Average Joe Cyclist Guide:
How to Buy the
Best Electric Bike

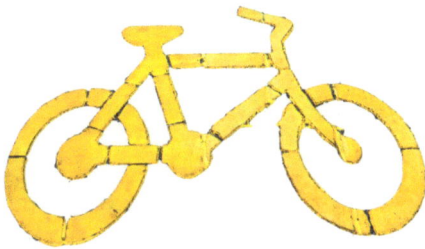

Published by Brave New World Publishing

© 2015 Joe Goodwill
ISBN: 978-0-9878986-8-5

www.averagejoecyclist.com

If you find this guide useful, you might also like:
Average Joe Cyclist Bike Buyers Guide

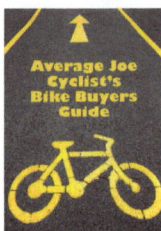

and
**Extraordinary Recipes:
How We Lost Weight by Eating Well**

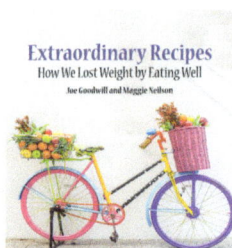

See all buying options in our online shop at
http://averagejoecyclist.com/shop/

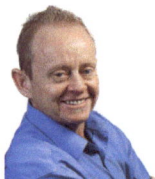

And see our cycling blog,
www.averagejoecyclist.com,
which has tons of free information

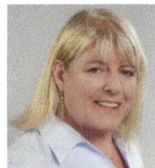

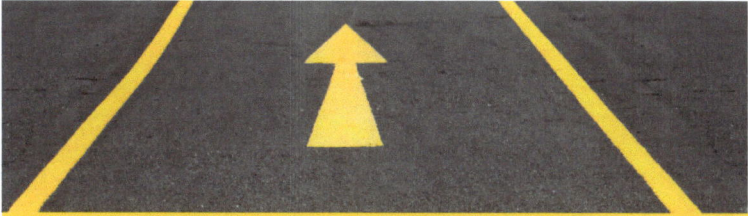

Average Joe Cyclist Guide:
How to Buy the
Best Electric Bike

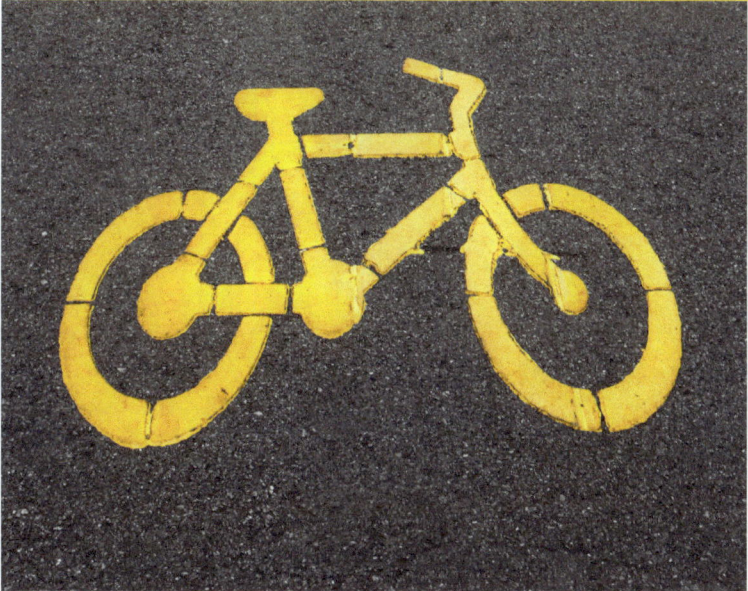

Table of Contents

Introduction

Most people don't spend a couple of thousand dollars without thinking carefully about their purchase. Electric bikes are expensive, high-technology machines – they are not something anyone should buy on the spur of the moment.

Research is required to ensure you spend your hard-earned money wisely and get years of savings, transport and good health from your purchase.

This is especially the case today, as more and more cheap electric bikes are flooding the market, making decisions all the more complicated. Do you buy cheap and hope for the best, or sink a lot of money into a really high-end, quality bike? It is definitely not a one-size-fits-all situation. A 100-pound woman commuting 20 miles a day on flat ground in a moderate climate needs a different electric bike than a 350-pound man commuting 40 miles a day on hilly ground in a snowy city. The bottom line is that there is no such thing as "the perfect electric bike." You could buy the most expensive electric bike in the world, but if it didn't suit your needs, it would not be the right electric bike for you.

The bike that best meets your individual needs is the best electric bicycle for you, and this book will help you figure out which bike that is.

I have used electric bikes for many years. I also belong to several cycling organizations, do volunteer work to promote cycling, run an electric bike meet-up group, and write several bike blogs, including my own (www.averagejoecyclist.com). Over the years, through personal experience and through talking to many different people, I have learned a great deal about electric bikes, and I want to pass that knowledge on to others. A good electric bike is not cheap, but if you buy the right one, it could save you a lot of money, improve your health and generally change your life for the better – so it's worth investing a little time to read this book and make sure you buy the right electric bike for your needs.

No matter who you are or what your needs are, this book includes all the information you need to make a wise decision when you buy your electric bike.

Even though electric bikes are high tech machines, you don't need to worry if you're not a techie genius. I have made sure that all the information in this book is down-to-earth: you won't need a degree in electrical engineering to understand all you need to know.

What I have done is give you an overview of the relevant technology, and then bottom lined it down to the nugget that the average buyer needs to know when choosing an electric bike. You can choose to assimilate all of the technology, or just use the bottom line to guide you.

Happy cycling!

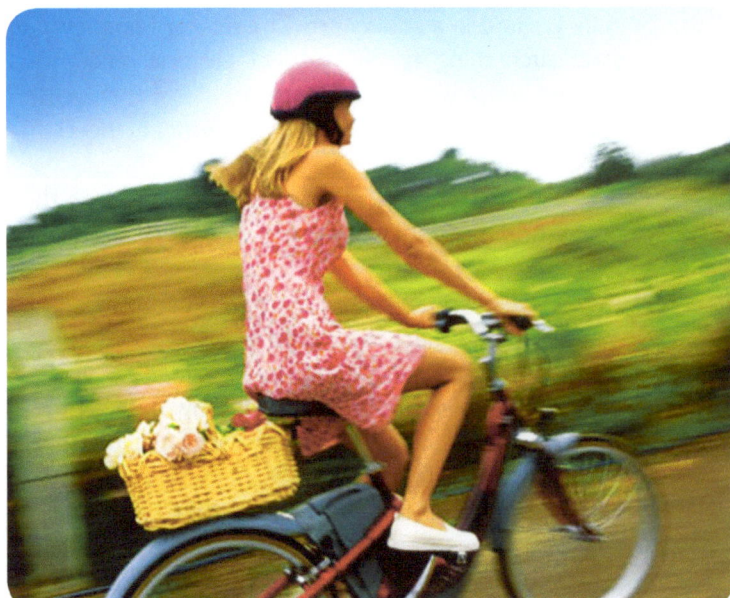

Electric Bikes are for Everyone!

As gas prices and obesity skyrocket, more and more people are looking for creative, sustainable alternatives for their transport needs – and more and more people are seeing the incredibly exciting potential of electric bikes. Electric bikes make cycling possible for average people – not just the lean, young, fit minority. As a result, they offer almost everyone a way to travel without gas and get fit at the same time – at a cost that is almost ludicrously cheap compared to cars. No wonder the popularity of electric bikes is soaring!

In 2010, 27 million electric bikes were sold; by 2011, that number had grown to 30 million. Admittedly, 28 million of those were in China, but the European market grew by 20%, to reach 1.2 million electric bikes. Today, electric bikes are the most successful mass-produced electric vehicles in the world.

It is predicted that by 2025, sales of electric bikes will reach 90 million per year – so if you're interested in buying an electric bike, you are not alone.

There are now so many good electric bikes available that almost anyone can be a cyclist. I use my own electric bike all the time, cycling to places I could never reach on a regular bike – and routinely passing people half my age as I pedal uphill. And because my bike looks just like a regular bike, and the motor is completely silent, they think I'm doing it on my own steam! I love it, because it makes me feel like a bionic man. I once almost killed a young guy after passing him effortlessly on my BionX bike. He chased me for miles, apparently determined not to let someone older than his father leave him in the dust. Eventually I glanced back and noticed the poor guy was about three heartbeats away from cardiac failure, so I let him pass me. I'm out there to travel and have fun, not to kill people!

Electric bikes blend muscle and machine into a better, faster, stronger you – and isn't that what we all want?

Electric bikes get you places far faster than a regular bike, with less sweat. For example, most Americans live less than five miles from their place of work. On an electric bike, zipping right by the traffic jams, this distance can be covered in 20 to 30 minutes. When traffic is heavy, this kind of commute is often faster than could be achieved on a regular bike or in a car. And the bonus is that electric bikes also make you fitter:

Research has shown that the average person who buys an electric bike gets fitter than the average person who buys a regular bike.

This is because people who buy electric bikes actually use them to get around. Hills and distance are not a deterrent when your electric bike makes you four times stronger than you usually are. It's like being the Incredible Hulk, only without the rage, greenness and mass destruction. And you can get your exercise during the dead time you previously wasted on commuting by car or transit.

I am passionate about electric bikes because they make cycling available to almost everyone – including those of us who are past 50, or have bad knees, or weak hearts, or who are carrying an extra 5 or 50 or 150 pounds. Electric bikes help everyone to cycle, so there are more bicycles and fewer cars. And the more cyclists there are, the safer it is to cycle: motorists are more likely to notice and respect cyclists when their numbers are greater. That explains why far fewer cyclists are killed in Europe than in North America, even though the number of cyclists in Europe is far greater. There are some cycling purists who accuse cyclists on electric bikes of "cheating," but I believe they should rather feel grateful that electric cyclists are helping to keep all cyclists safer, simply by swelling the numbers.

I also love electric bikes because I truly believe they are a move in the direction of saving our beloved planet for the next generation; I rejoice every time I see someone out shopping on an electric bike, instead of burning up the ozone with an unnecessary SUV. I've been using electric bikes for more than a decade now, and I have the satisfaction of knowing that I have massively decreased my own contribution to the destruction of the planet that my children will inherit.

Electric bikes provide the best of all worlds: you get to exercise; you get to have fun and feel like a super hero; you can travel efficiently, cheaply and quickly; and almost everyone can use them, as they come in regular bikes, recumbent and trikes (three-wheeled cycles).

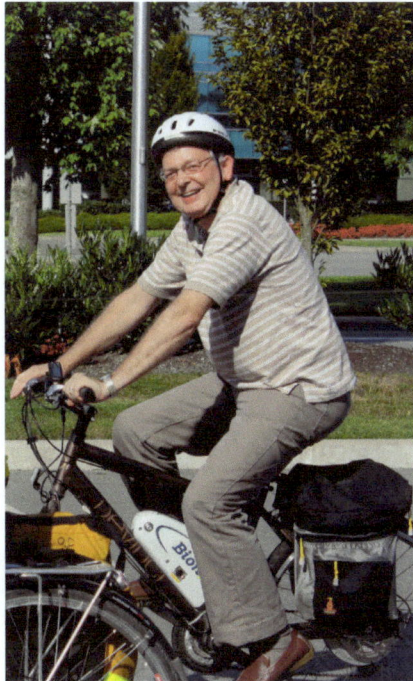

What are Electric Bikes?

Electric bikes are essentially very simple, consisting of four parts:

- bike
- battery
- controller
- motor

The simplicity of electric bikes means that some users will be able to service these bikes themselves, and even upgrade them or make them faster. (If you're interested in this, I recommend Matthew Slinn's book, *Build your own Electric Bicycle*.) However, the average user does not have to know how they work – you just need to be able to pedal a bike. The controls for electric assistance are very simple to use.

Electric bikes bring together human and electrical power by assisting you with pedaling, so they are a hybrid of human and electric power. Even though they employ some non-human power, electric bikes are different from motorbikes, in that:

- Almost all of them can be pedaled. In fact, the law often requires that the pedals stay on the bike, even if you don't use them all the time, in order for them to continue to be classified as bikes. However, most of them will move when you are not pedaling. It's just that most are not designed to be used that way, so you will wear the battery down very fast if you don't pedal.
- Usually the power and speed of electric bikes is limited by law. This is actually a good thing in one way: it enables most electric bikes to be exempt

from vehicle registration and the plethora of laws that are associated with this. For example, in the United States some states allow all bikes with motors under 750 W peak power to be exempt from vehicle registration. However, some US states don't allow electric bikes at all. On the other hand, in Europe an electric bike must have no more than 250 W maximum continuous power and weigh less than 88 pounds in order to be exempt from vehicle registration. In Canada, electric bikes must be fitted with pedals in order to be treated as bikes and be exempt from motor vehicle registration and regulations.

- Electric bikes are almost always allowed to use bike lanes and routes, which of course enables the rider to zip by traffic!

Electric bikes are still relatively new in the West, but they are a rapidly growing phenomenon. In China, they already outnumber cars by four to one. I believe that this will be echoed in the West one day, although I am not sure if it will be in my lifetime. I hope so.

Certainly all the demographic trends are favorable: fewer and fewer young people are getting drivers' licenses and buying cars. They are becoming what is known as the "Smart Generation" or the "Creative Class" – young people who would rather spend their money on smart phones, bikes and other gadgets, and who don't choose to waste hours of their day driving a car.

For example, a study by the Frontier Group in 2012 found that annual miles traveled by car among people aged 16 to 34 dropped by 23% in the time period 2001 to 2009. At the same time, their number of bike trips rose by 24% in the same time periods. And the modern world is catering to that trend. Between 1874 and 2011, the USA built a total of 62 protected, separated bike lanes. But in the year 2012, US cities built another 40 – almost doubling in one year the number of bike lanes that had taken 137 years to build.

Most electric bikes are powered by electricity

from a regular power source, such as you might use for your toaster or your razor. More and more places are incorporating electric bike and car charging stations in their new buildings. In the meantime, you can usually plug your bike battery in almost anywhere to charge while you are working, shopping or visiting. I have often plugged mine in to charge under a seat in a waiting room. Note that pedaling does not charge the battery (unlike hybrid cars, where the engine charges the battery).

What kind of battery does an electric bike use?

A wide range of commercial batteries is available, and this subject is discussed in a later chapter. Note that car batteries are the worst choice.

How much do electric bikes cost?

There is a massive variation, from a few hundred dollars right up to $12,000, and even beyond. Expect to pay upwards of $1,000 for a good electric bike. Quality costs money, and you get what you pay for. Trite, but true. There is also an excellent chance of getting a good deal second hand, if you know what you are doing.

How much do electric bikes weigh?

Electric bikes usually weigh between 55 and 88 pounds. Regular bikes weigh in between about 18 and 30 pounds. However, there are electric bikes that way as little as around 30 pounds.

How fast do electric bikes go?

Electric bikes usually only travel at up to about 20 miles per hour, but it is possible to make them faster. Gravity helps too! And as with regular bikes, the less you weigh, the faster you are likely to go. However, unlike with regular bikes, you can load up with a lot of luggage and still go at a good speed.

How far do electric bikes go?

Essentially they go until both the battery and your legs give out. Most batteries are only designed to have a range of about 20 miles, but this can be improved on with better batteries and by carrying extra batteries. Manufacturers are constantly working on improving the range. Currently there are electric bikes on sale that purport to be capable of up to a hundred miles on one battery charge. Bear in mind that sales claims may be exaggerated. Also, range depends on a wide variety of factors, including rider weight, how much you pedal, and terrain.

How long will the battery last?

Most will last for several years. They are rated for battery cycles, so the frequency with which you use them will have an impact. However, if you let your battery lie idle for several months, it may die – like humans, they need some exercise. If you plan to stop cycling during winter, put your charger on a timer, so that the battery gets about 30 minutes of charging per week. This will usually prevent it from dying on you.

Do you have to pedal an electric bike?

Most electric bikes will allow you to go without pedaling at all. Of course, this means you won't get fit, and you will use up the battery very quickly. Some electric bikes (called pedelecs) require you to pedal before power is generated by the motor. Most electric bike users prefer to pedal because they enjoy cycling and want to get fit and burn calories, and because they want to save the battery for the uphill bits, or for when they get very tired. But of course, you can use your own bike any way you like.

Why use an electric bike instead of a regular bike?

It is true that regular bikes are the most efficient transport machines in the world. However, electric bikes enable cycling without sweating, they are faster, they make it MUCH easier to go up hills, they enable you to carry more luggage, they tend to be safer as it is easier to keep up with traffic, and the power source can be used for powerful lights and horns. Finally, electric bikes make cycling possible for people who are older, or who have a variety of physical challenges. In short they combine the ease of motorized transport with the fun of a bicycle. They are also excellent for young, healthy people who have an extremely long and difficult commute, and for people towing a load.

Are electric bikes bad for the environment?

No, they are great for the environment. They cause far less pollution than cars. And in fact emissions for electric power production are lower than for human power. (Lemire-Elmore, 2004) Human emissions include carbon dioxide. And in order for us to produce power we have to eat, and these days, our food has usually been shipped half way around the world, meaning that every burger you eat has left a trail of emissions in its wake.

14 Reasons to Get an Electric Bike

In case you're still wondering if an electric bike is the right choice for you, consider the following 14 excellent reasons to get an electric bike. I wanted to make this a list of 10, but there are just so many reasons to get an electric bike that I could not stop at 10.

Health and Fitness

You'd think a regular bike would keep you fitter than an electric bike – and you'd be right, if you rode the regular bike as much as you rode the electric bike. But trust me, the average cyclist just will not ride a regular bike as much as an electric bike. Would I ride my regular bike up the steep hill I live on just to buy a bottle of wine or a loaf of bread? Would I ride it into a howling head wind? Would I ride it when I'm hauling 50 pounds? Not likely – I'd take my wife's car. Sadly, this would not make me fitter. But my electric bike will.

And I'm not the only one – the latest research shows a third of regular bikes are used less than 25 times a year, with 46% being used a paltry once or twice a week. However, 30% of people with electric bikes use them at least once a day, and a whopping 81% ride their bikes at least once a week. Bottom line, as verified by the Transport Research Laboratory in the United Kingdom: electric bikes are used at least twice as often as regular bikes. And as we all know from the workout machines that serve as laundry dryers in basements all over this great continent of ours, machines only make you fit if you actually use them.

On a personal note, my electric bike has made it possible for me to live car-free, and for most people, that is just not possible on a regular bike. I do most of my every-day commuting on my electric bike. So despite the fact that I am a strong cyclist and often have a lot of fun on my regular bikes, my very high level of fitness is mainly the result of my electric bike, not my regular bikes.

All of the bikes discussed in this book employ a combination of pedaling and electric assistance. The exercise you will get on your electric bike is good, low-intensity cardio exercise, often of long duration. For example, commuting to work on an electric bike might provide you with 30 to 60 minutes of low-intensity cardio, twice a day, five days a week – for a possible total of 12 hours per week of exercise. This adds up to a whopping amount of exercise done and calories burned – all in the time you would normally have done nothing but grow old and fat while trapped in traffic in your car.

While the motor of your electric bike will help you out, you will still be getting regular, consistent exercise on your electric bike – and all doctors agree that regular, consistent exercise is key to good cardiovascular, general and mental health.

Bottom line: Deciding to buy an electric bike is not just a transport decision – it's a decision to enrich the quality and length of your life by getting healthier and fitter.

Weight Loss

Commuting by electric bike is an excellent way to lose weight. In general, cycling is a great way to burn calories, because you're so focused on the journey and the fun that you can easily spend several hours exercising.

You burn a lot of calories on an electric bike, because although you have assistance, you are also moving a heavier bike. It doesn't completely balance out, but according to actual tests done by an engineer (see p. 30), you can expect to burn around 80% as many calories on your electric bike as you would on a regular bike.

So here is a calculation to help you work out how many calories you burn in an hour on an electric bike, cycling at an easy pace:

1. Start with your weight in pounds, e.g. 250 pounds
2. Divide this by 2.2 to give you your weight in kg, in this case, 113.6 kg
3. Multiply 113.6 by 6, to give you 632 calories per hour on a regular bike at an easy pace
4. Multiply 632 by 80%, to allow for the help from your electric bike
5. … equals 505 calories burned in 1 hour

So if you weigh 250 pounds and you're spending 2 hours per day, five days a week, commuting on your electric bike, you are burning an extra 2,090 extra calories every week. If you do this 49 weeks per year (allowing for 3 weeks' vacation), you're burning 247,450 extra calories per year. You have to burn 3,500 calories to lose a pound – which means that switching from a car to an electric bike could result in a weight loss of about 70 pounds in one year. Not to mention that even after you park your electric bike in your garage you continue to burn more calories, because you have revved up your metabolism by cycling.

My own experience bears this out. I have spent my entire life trying not to be fat. However, my body has done its utmost to stay fat. I have never managed to turn the tide in that battle – until ten years ago, when I started doing most of my commuting on an electric bike. How did the electric bike turn the tide? In a nutshell, it keeps me honest about exercise. I can't tell you how many times I've resolved to hit the gym five times a week, or swim twice a week, or get back into soccer. Usually I do it for a few weeks and then … I stop. On the other hand, since I resolved to give up my car and commute by electric bike, exercise just inevitably happens. I have to get to work, and once I'm there, I have to get back.

Thanks to my electric bike I am now down 60 pounds, and my wife actually referred to my body the other day as "wiry". Wow – I never thought I'd ever hear the word "wiry" applied to me!

Admittedly, my weight loss is also due to the very healthy (but delicious) eating plan that my wife and I follow.

We developed healthy recipes based on the various diets we tried. Our idea was to enjoy eating but still lose weight. We did, and so we have published a recipe book based on our wholesome but delicious recipes. You can buy it from our website shop (http://averagejoecyclist.com/shop/), or direct from Amazon.

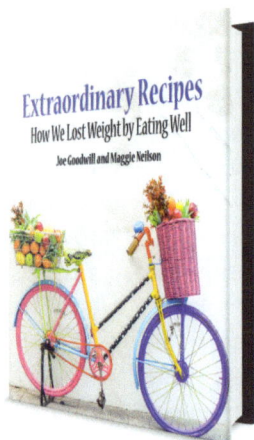

Faster Travel

This is one of my favorite fun facts: although modern cars can achieve speeds up to 50 times greater than cars at the turn of the twentieth century, average car speed in traffic has not increased at all. I find that mildly hilarious. The reason is obvious to anyone who has ever sat in traffic gridlock: it doesn't help to have a car that is capable of traveling at 200 miles per hour, if the 50,000 gridlocked cars in front of you are managing a death-defying ten miles per hour.

On your electric bike you will be able to cycle faster than the average cyclist, yet still use the cycle routes that cars and motorcycles cannot use. As a result, you may well find that your electric bike is your fastest way to get to work.

Personally I have never had a single commute on my electric bike where I did not at some point whiz past a car as if it was standing still. Usually I pass hundreds of almost stationary cars. Every time I drive past a car I am reminded of how much I loath the experience of driving a car: locked in a tin can, getting mad at other drivers and having them get mad at me. When I am forced to drive I find myself staring wistfully at the cyclists whizzing past me, obviously full of joy and exercise-induced endorphins, and find myself seriously questioning one of the fundamental myths of modern society: the notion that the motor car represents convenience and freedom.

As I inch along in traffic gridlock, all I can think is: "HOW exactly is this convenience and freedom?"

No Sweat

Sweat is an important issue if you're cycling to work, and most people aren't lucky enough to have shower facilities at the office. People sweat less on electric bikes, because they don't have to pedal as hard, and because the higher speed means there is more wind to keep you cool. I loved this story, told by a committed cyclist who somewhat grudgingly tried out an electric bike:

> "I changed my tune about electric bikes after my first long commute. I had mounted Schwinn's top-of-the-line Tailwind e-bike in leafy Brooklyn, dubious of the proposition of a battery-powered bicycle. Cyclists, after all, ride to exercise. This seemed like cheating. Seven miles later, by the time I got to Times Square, it dawned on me. The e-bike isn't about exercise, strictly. It's about commuting. The bike's electric motor helped me climb up to the Brooklyn Bridge, and then ascend a long incline from the Hudson River to the traffic-choked heart of Manhattan. The Tailwind transformed a normally sweaty bike commute into a pleasant, energizing spin. Indeed, I had given up on bike commuting to work because the ride left me drenched, and with no shower at work, it was a no go. The e-bike made bike commuting possible again." (Adam Aston, "The Schwinn Tailwind: An E-bike for Commuters", Bloomberg Business Week, http://www.businessweek.com/innovate/content/mar2009/id20090330_206308.htm)

Safety

"Let me tell you what I think of bicycling. I think it has done more to emancipate women than anything else in the world. It gives women a feeling of freedom and self-reliance. I stand and rejoice every time I see a woman ride by on a wheel ... the picture of free, untrammeled womanhood." (Susan B. Anthony, 1820-1906, abolitionist and leader of the American women's suffrage movement.)

It is well known that male cyclists outnumber female cyclists pretty much everywhere. Research indicates this has much to do with safety: cycling is perceived as unsafe, and because of this, many women don't want to cycle (perhaps because of a sense of responsibility towards the many people that most women take care of). This is very unfortunate, not least because bike riding is so liberating (as Susan B. Anthony noticed a long time ago).

In this respect, I have a lot of hope for the potential of electric bikes. An electric bike is less dangerous than a regular bike. As soon as you start riding one, you will notice how the ability to quickly accelerate, and to occasionally keep up with motorized traffic, both help to keep you out of danger. You are less likely to be rear ended because motorists have more time to see you. Intersections are the scene of most collisions, and the fast acceleration of electric bikes gets you out of the danger zone faster. The fewer cars have to overtake you, the safer you are. Plus, because you have power to help you go up hills, you don't have the temptation to go downhill at high speeds to get your speed up for the upcoming ascent – definitely a useful safety feature. Also, cyclists on electric bikes are more likely to stop at stop signs and red lights, because they have the power to easily pull off again.

Also, the power source on electric bike is often used to power lights and horns. You can have a bike light that is 20 times stronger than a regular bike light, which of course makes you much more visible and hence much safer.

In case you're reading this and thinking that nothing

will make bikes safer than cars, consider this: cars are the number one killer of people under 35 in the USA (including children). The danger posed by cars is so extreme that some people have suggested that cars should carry warning labels, just as cigarettes do.

Easy Hill Climbing

Most electric cyclists remember the first time they ever tackled a serious hill. It's a wonderful moment, a sudden feeling of almost superhuman ability. Electric bikes flatten hills out, so that the cyclist does not have to dread them. Depending on the power of your bike, you may still have to put in a fair amount of effort – but it will be much less than when doing hills without an electric assist. As an older cyclist, when I first started cycling I often had to resort to the embarrassing get-off-and-push maneuver, but once I got an electric bike that became a thing of the past. Even in the incredibly hilly city in which I live, I never have to dismount and push.

Save Money

Most people need some form of transport. In the Western world this is often a private car, occupied most of the time by just one person. The cost of this luxury is enormous, and in fact cars are usually the second biggest expense in most people's budgets (after housing). Imagine the vacations you could afford if you could massively reduce this enormous expense. An electric bike will enable you to be completely or partly car-free, which will enable enormous savings.

It is true that buying an electric bike will cost you more than buying a regular bike. Your upkeep costs will be much the same as for a regular bike, but for electric bikes, an extra expense comes from battery depreciation – they don't last forever, and the replacement cost for a good battery is usually pretty high. Thus, all in all, electric bikes are definitely more expensive to run than regular bikes.

However, once the running costs of electric bikes are compared to cars or even transit, the picture is much brighter. Electric bikes are definitely the most fuel-efficient mode of transport in everyday use. In fact, some people have done the math to prove that electric bikes are more fuel-efficient than humans. One thing is for sure: it is cheaper to run my electric bike than to run a car. I don't even notice the cost of recharging my battery on my electric bill – it's basically negligible. No one can say that about the cost of gas for a car. And of course I recharge the battery at work, at negligible cost to my employer.

This is a very different scenario from the years of expensive car-owning I have gone through. Most of us are seduced by the ads that tell us that a shiny new car will cost us just a couple of hundred dollars a month. However, this does not factor in all of the following costs:

- A high cost price, no matter how you pay it. You could buy the most expensive electric bike on the planet, and it would still only cost about half the price of the cheapest new car. My own high-end electric bike cost 10% of what my last car cost (around $3,000 for the bike and $30,000 for the car).
- High insurance costs
- Constantly increasing gas prices
- High and sometimes crippling repair charges (on my last car, just replacing the clutch cost $2,000 – I could have bought a very good electric bike for that price.)
- High maintenance charges for services and oil changes

Young people in particular have to pay very high vehicle insurance prices, so they could save thousands of dollars and get around more quickly in cities by choosing an electric bike. In 2010 it was calculated that the running costs of a car are 60 times the running cost of an electric bike – and the cost of running cars is climbing steeply due to the relentlessly rising cost of gas.

Urban cities are becoming more and more congested

and difficult to navigate in cars. On an electric bike, you move around quickly and cheaply, and park for free. So you will also avoid the cost of parking tickets.

For most people the thought of surviving without a personal car is daunting, and many people believe it is entirely impossible. However, when an electric bike is combined with transit and/or car hire, or co-op car schemes, or taxis, it becomes quite easy. Check to see what options are available in your area. For example, renting a car once a month for a day of shopping would cost just a tiny fraction of what it costs to own a car all the time.

Motorized, but no Red Tape

In most jurisdictions electric bikes are regarded as regular bicycles, so you are not forced to get a license, or to pay taxes and insurance. You cannot be convicted for cycling under the influence of alcohol, either (although it is NOT a good idea to drink and cycle). You can take out insurance on your bike, and for third-party liability, and personally I would recommend it. But unlike almost everything to do with cars, it's optional.

Because electric bikes are categorized as bicycles, they can be ridden in bike lanes and on bike routes, giving riders a huge advantage over cars.

Note: you should be aware of the prevailing legislation in your own country, as there are some differences. For example, speed limits and power limitations are different in different countries.

Saving the World,
One Commute at a Time ...

"Every time I see an adult on a bicycle, I no longer despair for the future of the human race."
(H.G. Wells, novelist)

As a parent and grandparent, I am very happy to be reducing

my carbon footprint by riding an electric bike most of the time. Every time I do a trip on my electric bike instead of a car, I feel like a green warrior, doing my tiny bit to preserve the planet for the upcoming generations.

Of course, we live in a society that has been structured around motorized transport. This makes it close to impossible to avoid cars completely – for example, I cannot take my daughters to horse camp on a bicycle, because getting there involves 50 miles of highway, and I can't really see any of my kids sitting on my cross bar for that long.

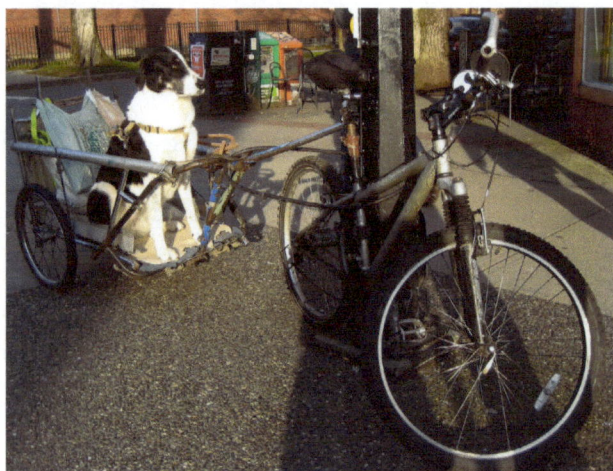

On the other hand, there are many situations in which one might think one needs a car, but really doesn't. For example, I saw a bike parked outside a local coffee bar the other day. The bike had a home-made trailer attached, and the trailer contained a large dog and a pile of shopping. Clearly the owner of that bike did not let the fact that he had to transport a dog and groceries deter him from using a bike. And that was just a regular bike, not even an electric bike. Sights like that make me resolve to reduce my dependency on cars even more.

I have also noticed an increasing number of parents using electric bikes to get their children to school. The extra weight of the child in a bike seat or trailer is offset by the power of the engine.

Average Joe Cyclist Guide

It is true that there are some inefficiencies in the production and distribution of electricity. However, the impact on the environment per mile of an electric bike remains negligible compared to the impact of a car. In fact, the amount of electricity required to run an electric bike is so low that it is feasible that in the future we will be able to recharge them with home-based solar power units. This would never suffice for the massive energy needs of a car.

It is surprising but true that electric bike power actually has less impact on the environment than human power.

This surprised me, as I assumed that I have zero emissions (apart from the usual biological functions). However, once one factors in all the energy and emissions that comprise our food chain, it appears that producing human energy in a person eating a typical Western diet does in fact result in significant emissions – up to five times as much as result from producing and running an electric bike. (Remember that in order for us to have enough energy to ride a regular bike or walk, an entire chain of activities is required, including farming, transport, refrigeration and cooking.) In short, human power is not as green as one might think, while the electric bike is the greenest, most efficient transport mode we have.

Escape Gas Dependency

"Those who wish to control their own lives and move beyond existence as mere clients and consumers – those people ride a bike." (Wolfgang Sachs, of the Wuppertal Institute for Climate, Environment and Energy and the former Chairman of Greenpeace, Germany)

The horrific BP oil spill in 2010 showed us that the gas on which we all depend is a very vulnerable commodity. And soaring prices constantly remind us that gas is a finite resource. But at the same time, over 90% of Americans still commute by car, and 77% of those drivers commute ALONE in their vehicles. We are devouring our expensive oil supplies like they will last forever – but they WON'T. Of course not everyone is going to stop driving cars completely – I know I haven't. But if a lot more of us use an electric bike at least some of the time, we can certainly reduce oil consumption, and help to make our oil last longer.

No More Parking Problems

You can park 20 bikes in the space it takes to park one car. Wherever I go, I can park my electric bike for free, usually right outside my destination. This ease of parking is one important reason why electric bikes often get travelers to their destination even faster than cars – the electric bike rider is already in the building, while the motorist is still driving around in frustrating circles, trying to find somewhere to (expensively) park their car.

Stop Supporting Terrorists

I came across this fascinating account by a man called Bryan A. Thompson. He owns a V8 Corvette, but has switched to using an electric bike for most of his travelling. Here he explains why:

"Recent attacks against my country culminating in the Sept. 11, 2001 tragedy have revealed that the folks that sell Americans more oil than any other country also sponsored (and largely provided) the terrorists responsible for those attacks. That country is Saudi Arabia. Unfortunately, because of America's dependence on oil, we have shown reluctance to pursue these terrorists into Saudi Arabia. When I learned of the Saudi's sponsorship of the terrorists responsible for killing close to 7000 Americans, I decided to do everything I could to keep as much money out of their hands as possible. It may not be much, but I've reduced my oil consumption by at least 40% – a level sustainable without Saudi oil." (http://www.batee.com/projects/offgrid/ebike/lafree/review.shtml)

Stress Relief and Feel-Good Factor

"When the spirits are low, when the day appears dark, when work becomes monotonous, when hope hardly seems worth having, just mount a bicycle and go out for a spin down the road, without thought of anything but the ride you are taking." (Arthur Conan Doyle)

Riding a bike makes you feel good. Studies have shown that people who cycle to work have the highest levels of satisfaction with their commute (followed closely by walkers). My own experience bears this out. As a cyclist, the best part of my workday is usually my commute. It invigorates me in the morning and de-stresses me in the evening. Researchers have concluded that the answer to commuter stress is not to build bigger, faster highways, but rather to provide safer bikeways so that people can get to work under their own power. Research shows that exercise can combat depression at least as effectively as (probably harmful) medications.

Also, it's a scientific fact that the more time we spend in the sunshine, the better we feel. Biking to work makes sure you spend some time outdoors, every day. The light inside is about 300 lux, while the light outside, even on an overcast day, is over 1,000 lux. All this light boosts your levels of the feel-good hormone, serotonin.

"Exercising outside exposes you to daylight," explains Professor Jim Horne from Loughborough University's Sleep Research Centre. "This helps get your circadian rhythm back in sync and rids your body of cortisol, the stress hormone that can prevent deep, regenerative sleep."

When I bike to work I arrive feeling fresh, energized and happy. (Which is very different from the way I used to feel when I would drive to work, and had to deal with traffic and road rage.) When I bike home, I can literally feel the stress falling off me with every passing mile, until I arrive home feeling rejuvenated and ready to enjoy my evening. Cycling on an electric bike is sufficiently brisk exercise that it raises endorphin levels, causing me to quite often break out into raucous singing while cycling! You don't have to go this far, but I promise you, riding an electric bike will make you feel great.

Work on your Tan while Commuting

One of the things I have discovered about cycle commuting is that it's an excellent way to tan. I was lying in a pool at a water park the other day, and noticed that I was the brownest Caucasian person there – just purely because I commute by bike. And it's a healthy tan, because I acquire it very slowly. If you think about it, cycle commuting usually means that you are out in the sun in the early morning and the late afternoon, which are the best times to slowly acquire a deep, healthy tan.

This may sound like a frivolous reason, but I think most people will relate. Now that I am middle-aged, I am very happy to be strong, toned, tanned and fit – I think it vastly increases my chances of retaining the interest of my lovely wife. And I wouldn't be like this if I spent most of my commuting time sitting on my spreading butt in a car, exercising nothing but my wrists and my right toe, and tanning nothing but my left elbow.

Electric Bikes and Good Health

Cardiovascular Health

There are countless stories of electric bikes turning people's health around. I used to cycle commute many years ago, but I stopped when I had a cardiovascular health scare. I missed cycling, and finally I got my cardiologist to agree to my cycling IF I used an electric assist to make sure I did not over-do things. I had my trusty Devinci hybrid commuter retrofitted with a BionX electric bike kit, and soon I was off and pedaling.

After just over a year of cycling with an electric bike, I was ready to go back to regular biking, and thanks to all the exercise, my health problems were just a memory. Ten years on, the cardiologist can find no trace of the plaque he detected in the arteries in my neck – so cycling has most likely saved me from having a stroke, by literally blowing out the plaque that had accumulated.

It is a known fact that exercise can reverse early stage cardiovascular disease, and I am the living proof that this can be done on an electric bike.

Even though I am now in excellent health, I still use my electric bike to get to work, because I have a massive hill to get over. The difference between me and my co-workers who also cycle to work: I do it EVERY day, while they are all too often daunted by the giant hill, so they drive instead. Electric bikes make it possible for me to cycle commute day after day, every day.

I use a Polar heart rate monitor to keep a check on how much exercise I get on my electric bike. This monitor shows me clearly that every time I ride my electric bike, I am within the optimal zone for cardiovascular conditioning for most of the ride. I am not at the high end, more at the low to medium level of conditioning. But as I sustain this for an hour and a half, it is ideal cardiovascular exercise. It keeps me in shape without exhausting me.

Back Problems

My wife Maggie had a similarly life-changing experience. A lifelong athlete and runner, she was stopped in her tracks at the age of 47 by a sudden back problem. While she waited for surgery to remove a cyst in her back, it became impossible for her to exercise, and eventually she could not even put on her own shoes. Finally she had surgery and her mobility was restored. Her doctor recommended cycling instead of running, because it is lower impact. But she was nervous because it had been many years since she rode a bike. I offered her the use of my electric bike. Now she says:

"The only thing that made me feel confident enough to get back on a bike was being able to ease into it with the electric bike. I loved it – it made me feel safe from injuring myself as I rehabilitated!"

After months of cycling on an electric bike, Maggie was fit and strong enough to transition to a regular bike on the weekends. These days she cycles to and from work on a regular bike, a round trip of 20 miles (32 km), because her route is completely flat. But she still uses an electric bike for days when we are going to be biking up hills. She has written a lot of posts about her experiences as a female cyclist-commuter on my blog at http://averagejoecyclist. com/. See the Category called "Mrs. Average Joe Cyclist.

Knee Pain

Many people with knee pain have been able to continue cycling only because of electric bikes. Particularly useful for knee pain are electric bikes that offer a choice of levels of assistance, such as BionX electric bikes, which offer three levels of assistance. This enables cyclists to use higher levels of assistance when their knees start to hurt, and decrease assistance when they don't need it as much. Many people are able to go back to regular cycling after a few years of strengthening their knees with an electric bike.

Heart Attacks

People with very serious health conditions can also use electric bikes as part of their recovery. One of my blog readers, Tom Childs, told me that he had two almost fatal heart attacks, which were treated with a couple of titanium spring loaded tubes in his coronary artery. That's a pretty big deal, and most people would never exercise again. But Tom went right out and bought a BionX PL-250 for his Norco Rideau. Later, he upgraded to a Dahon Matrix folding bike with a BionX PL-350. He beat all the odds, and he got back in shape – all it took was the heart of a lion, coupled with some electric assistance.

Healthy Exercise for the Over Fifties

Electric bikes make cycling accessible for a much wider range of people, and that's a wonderful thing! Many people over 50 have health issues to deal with, such as knee problems. And as we age, we all lose some strength, unfortunately. But the added power of electric bikes makes it possible for almost anyone to travel by bike.

For example, I know a courageous woman in her sixties who cycles everywhere on her electric bike, commuting in all but the heaviest downpours in the soggy city she lives in. She told me this story:

"I was cycling into work the other morning, and this young fellow pulled up beside me at a light, took a look at my BionX and told me I was cheating! I looked at him and told him in no uncertain terms, 'Young man, I'm 60 years old. When you've got another 40 years on those legs of yours, come back and talk to me!' He was rather taken aback – I don't think he realized how old I was. Plus I hadn't had my coffee yet, so I'm afraid I was not in the mood to put up with nonsense!"

She sure told him!

How Many Calories are Burned Cycling on an Electric Bike?

I was amazed to see how many calories are burned cycling on a regular bike. I have often wondered about burning calories on an electric bike, because I sometimes use a regular bike and sometimes use an electric bike (I prefer the electric bike for very hilly routes and very long rides).

Well, I recently met a brilliant bike engineer – Ron Wensel. Ron has proved that you can burn almost as many calories on an electric bike as on a regular bike.

Ron Wensel and his son Claudio make Pedal Easy electric bikes

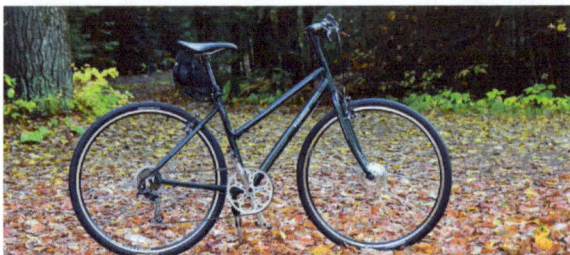

Ron was an engineer for decades, and he has used his experience to develop a very competitively-priced (around $1,500) range of lightweight, long-range electric bikes. The lightweight bikes are integrated with a small, high-efficiency battery and motor.

These very efficient electric bikes don't LOOK like electric bikes. The small, light battery is cunningly concealed in a saddle bag. The motor in the rear hub is so small that most people would not notice it. And the bikes are nicely specced with mid-range Shimano components. The frames are built to be super strong but lightweight.

Total weight of Pedal Easy electric bikes,
with battery and fenders, is as low as 28 pounds.

The electric assistance on these Pedal Easy bikes is controlled with a throttle. Because the bikes are so light, you can choose to use them as regular bikes (pedaling only) or on full throttle (no pedaling at all) – or somewhere in between.

Ron decided to develop these bikes four years ago, after he had survived four heart attacks. He wanted to keep on cycling, but his doctor warned him not to let his heart rate go over 140. With these electric bikes and his heart rate monitor, Ron can still do group bike rides and even go on long-distance biking vacations with his wife: he just wears a heart rate monitor, pedals the bike like a regular bike – and then uses the throttle whenever his heart rate is close to his "danger zone" of 140 beats per minute.

Keeping your heart rate under control with an electric bike

Ron took the electric bike on two one-hour rides over moderately hilly terrain. On the first ride he used throttle assist for the tougher parts. This enabled him to keep his heart rate under 140 (the red zone starts at 140).

A few days later Ron did the same bike ride on the same electric bike, but without throttle assist. His heart rate went well above 140 – sometimes even as high as 170 beats per minute. Fortunately, he survived this test.

Testing calories burned cycling on electric bikes

Ron's heart rate monitor supplied some very interesting information about calories burned on the two bike rides. He recorded both bike rides, with the number of calories burned on both rides. When Ron used the throttle assist to protect his heart, he burned up 444 calories during the one-hour bike ride. When he did the bike ride without throttle assist, he burned up 552 calories during the one-hour bike ride. This shows that using the electric bike resulted in burning only 20% less calories.

You can see pictures of the electronic records Ron made on my website at http://averagejoecyclist.com/how-many-calories-burned-cycling-electric-bike/. The graphics were too low-resolution to include in this book.

Burning 440 calories in an hour is a big deal – done regularly, this kind of calorie burn could result in significant weight loss.

I find this exciting for two reasons:

1. It shows that heart disease patients can use electric bikes to keep on cycling, while still following their doctor's orders about keeping their heart rate fairly low.
2. It shows that many calories are burned cycling on an electric bike.

How an Electric Bike Can Help to Come Back From an Injury

A while ago I suffered a bad injury that put me out of cycling for several months. Just before that injury I could cycle up to about 80 km a day and feel just fine. I was in training to do the Enbridge Ride to Conquer Cancer, and I was confident that I would soon be able to do it quite easily.

Then disaster struck, and my body was set back badly. For a long time all I concentrated on was getting back normal daily functions, because even the most simple things – like watching TV, showering and walking – were difficult. It was depressing as hell.

But I tried to focus on imagining myself back in the saddle, cycling mile after mile, strong and effortless, like the athlete I used to be.

And yes, I know I have never LOOKED much like a super athlete, but I sure have FELT like one, and I used to exercise much like I imagine real athletes exercise.

Finally, I was able to get back on my bike. BUT with a difference: to start out, I used my electric bike (a Devinci Sydney retrofitted with an excellent BionX kit, which you can read about here). This meant I could go through the motions of cycling, but use as much (or more to the point, as little) energy as I wanted. Even using the motor at full power, each bike ride exhausted me, and I would lie on the couch afterwards, feeling like I'd been sat on by an elephant, and then had to run away from a ferocious rhinoceros. Not fun, and I am sure I was no fun to be with, lying on the couch and whining loudly.

Nonetheless, I was happy and proud that I was at least

going through the motions – my legs were pumping my pedals in a motion that exactly resembled being a real cyclist, even if I was benefiting from a whole lot of help. My mood improved, just because I was getting out there and getting SOME exercise. And of course, I was getting to experience the joy of riding a bike – something I always find joyful, whether its on a regular bike or an electric bike, in the sunshine or in a monsoon-like rain storm.

I took my wife's advice and took it slow. Truth to tell, even I knew it was smart to take it slow.

I did not try to graduate to a regular bike until the rides on my electric bike ONLY made me feel as if I had been chased by an ELDERLY rhinoceros. Finally I got there, and I started interspersing my electric bike rides with regular bike rides.

On my very first ride on my regular bike, I was passed by an older man on an uphill. He gave me a huge smile and confided, "I don't usually PASS people." I looked at him in his full construction gear, including steel-toed boots, riding his rusty, ancient bike. I was riding my slick-looking racer, and was decked out in full, expensive cycling gear from head to toe. Regardless, he passed me with the greatest of ease.

Because I am a nice guy, I resisted the urge to shout: "I'm coming back from an injury!" Instead, I forced a smile through my teeth, said "Good for you!", and let him enjoy his moment of triumph. (I'll get him one day ...)

In short, it was a bit depressing at first. I could do 80 km with ease before, and now 10 km was tiring – and 20 km was killer. But I kept going, inching up my distances, trying to slowly improve without overdoing it.

After a few weeks, I finally started to ENJOY the rides on my regular bike. I found myself standing up in the pedals, feeling exhilarated, feeling like an athlete. It's absolutely the best feeling you can have with your clothes on.

Now I can feel my strength growing and my energy increasing. Every day I feel just a tiny bit stronger. And I can feel the joy of cycling rising in my heart again.

The point is, it's a process. Take it slow, listen to your body, but don't give up, and trust that you'll get there. Remember what bought you to cycling in the first place: the love of cycling. You still have that love, and you can and will enjoy it again.

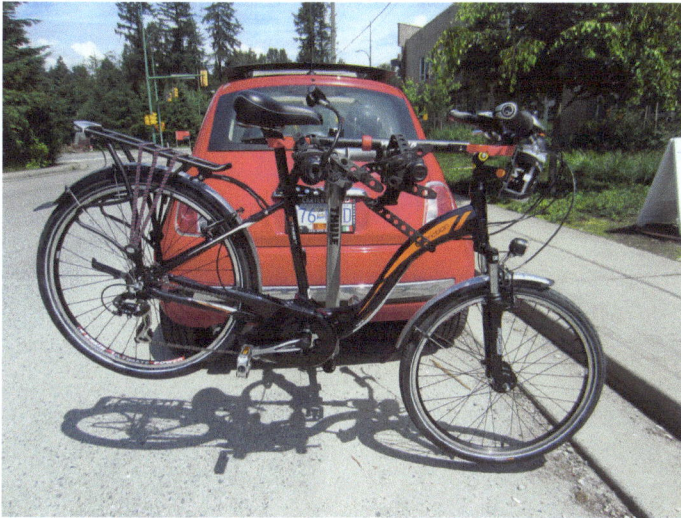

What are you waiting for? Buy yourself an electric bike and start getting into shape. Electric bikes can be transported on the smallest of cars. Here's an Emotion Street 650 on the back of a Fiat 500.

Electric Bikes and the Law: A Pretty Sweet Deal

Speed Limits

There are laws to control the speed of cars, and there are also laws to control the speed of electric bikes. But here's the weird part: while a teenager can go out and buy a car that can travel at triple the speed limit, most electric bikes are cleverly rigged so that even wise old seniors cannot exceed the speed limit. I find this bizarre, as a car doing 120 miles an hour can do a lot more damage than a bicycle doing 35 miles an hour. Yet for some reason, car drivers are trusted to be sensible and law-abiding, while electric cyclists are not. I have some theories about the reasons for this, but writing about them would put me at risk of sounding bitter, cynical and even demented, so I won't.

Suffice it to say that you should check the speed limit in your area, and try to stick to it. It won't be hard, as your bike won't let you go much faster (unless you are a computer genius who can figure out how to overcome the built-in restrictions on your electric bike).

I have to admit that I sometimes exceed the speed limit while travelling downhill – my legs and gravity make up for the fact that the assist stops working at 20 miles per hour, which is the speed limit in my part of the world.

Electric Bikes on Bike Paths

In most jurisdictions, electric bikes are allowed to use all routes designated for regular bicycles. Believe it or not, there are some cyclists who feel passionately that electric bikers should stay off cycle routes, and mix it up with cars instead. In my opinion, such cyclists are bitter and twisted, and do not represent the average cyclist, who tends to be a friendly, kind person who does not want other cyclists to die – even if they do need a bit of an assist to get up a hill.

I once did a blog post on this subject, and one of the commentators, Steven Luscher, really nailed the issue. He wrote:

"The bike vs. electric bike and e-scooter debate, with respect to who should be allowed to ride in what lane, and on what path, often centers around a formal analysis of vehicle shape, size, width, weight, and speed. To analyze the issue in this way is to miss the most important question of all, the answer to which should solely decide which type of vehicle should ride in the bike lane: is it vulnerable in traffic?

Vulnerability is what separates us from cars, vans, and trucks, and it is the banner under which we should all be able to rally. By "us," of course, I mean bikes, tandems, electric bikes, e-scooters, unicycles, Pedersens, prones, sociables, penny-farthings, recumbent trikes, and others; any vehicle whose physical limitations put its rider at risk of a fatal accident with a car, van, or truck in traffic.

I propose that we bury the hatchet over this debate; electrified or not, we are all equally at risk of a fatal accident in traffic. Our mutual vulnerability, coupled with our compassion for other human beings, should forever answer the question of whether to allow electric bikes in bike lanes and on bike paths: "yes."

To which I can only say, "Amen."

Pedal-free Option

In the USA and Canada, it is legal to have electric bikes that can go without any pedaling, usually using a throttle control. Examples are BionX and Pedego. These are illegal in most of the rest of the world, for reasons known only to lawmakers in their infinite wisdom.

On the other hand, in 2012 the Supreme Court of Canada ruled that as soon as you take the pedals off your electric bike, it is no longer a bike. It then falls into a gray area of being neither a motor vehicle nor a bike, and owners may be fined for not licensing them (as they don't belong to any category that exists for licensing, and therefore the owners cannot license them).

So in Canada it comes down to: you have to have pedals on your bike, even if they are purely decorative and you never actually use them. I'm glad I never followed the option of becoming a lawyer: clearly I am not smart enough to be one, because to me, some laws appear screamingly ludicrous.

Should Cyclists Obey the Traffic Laws?

One of the most controversial blog posts I ever did was on the issue of whether cyclists should slavishly follow all of the rules of the road. At the time I wrote it, my view was simple: yes, we should obey the law, to the letter, just as motorists are expected to do (although of course, in practice, most motorists do break the law, a lot). But as often happens on my blog, I got some interesting counter arguments from my erudite readers, and I ended up feeling a lot less certain.

Readers pointed out that the traffic laws are made and implemented with cars in mind. Therefore, some of the laws might not be applicable. For example, there are many times when it is perfectly safe for a cyclist to merely slow down at a Stop sign. Bikes are a lot slower than cars, after all. And there are times – such as on a steep uphill – when coming to a complete stop imposes a lot of extra work on a cyclist. Also, for the many cyclists who use clipless pedals, stopping completely requires unclipping, which many don't do, preferring to balance for a second or two. Of course (and I'm speaking from bitter experience here), that opens up the possibility of falling over sideways and hitting the sidewalk in spectacular fashion – which could be deadly if a bus is coming. And very unpleasant for the bus driver. In this situation, a rolling stop would actually be safer than a complete stop.

Also, from my own observation, there are places where there are wide sidewalks that are untouched by pedestrian feet, next to roads that are dangerous for cyclists because of traffic density and speed. In such situations, it is often safer for the cyclist (and less annoying for motorists) if the cyclist takes to the sidewalk. However, in most jurisdictions there is a blanket ban on this: it is always illegal for cyclists to mount the sidewalk, even if it's a no-brainer that it will save their lives and inconvenience no one. Personally, I have taken to using my discretion on this one. But I wouldn't advise anyone else, one way or the other – this is a case where you have to employ your own common sense and values.

That said, proof that traffic laws should be different for cyclists some of the time comes from jurisdictions that are considering allowing cyclists to roll through stop signs. Arizona is one such place – lawmakers argue that cyclists should be allowed to treat stop signs as yield signs, exercising discretion and only stopping if there is other traffic. Imagine that – a law that assumes cyclists have common sense and can maturely exercise discretion! This is the kind of thing that renews my faith in the universe.

Tips for Electric Bike Commuters

Extend your Range

One of the most important issues for every electric biker is range: how far will your electric bike take you before the battery runs out of charge? This can be a real problem – for example, I recall once sitting in a cafeteria at a hospital, drinking possibly the worst cup of coffee ever made, while inhaling disgusting hospital smells – all on a lovely sunny summer's day. The reason for this? My battery had run down, and there were a lot of uphills between the hospital and my home. So I sat in that restaurant sipping that horrible coffee and playing with my iPhone for an entire hour, waiting patiently for my battery to recharge …

There are better ways. I hate to admit that it took me years to figure this one out, but it did: if you're doing a long trip, CARRY A SPARE BATTERY! Yes, it really did take me years to figure this out. In my defense, spare batteries are not cheap – not if they're good batteries, anyway. But honestly, it's worth the outlay. With the power of your electric assist, you won't even feel the extra weight – and you will double your range. Simple, yet totally effective.

Of course, the range of electric bikes is constantly being improved by competing manufacturers, so if your commute is not too long, range may not be an issue. Personally I keep a spare charger at work, and simply let my battery recharge as I work, so that I have plenty of power to get me home.

All About Bike Lights

I shudder every time I see a cyclist dressed in black on an unlit bike on a dark night. I pray when I see a cyclist with very few lights towing a small child or baby. To me this is a no-brainer: be bright, be visible, and stay alive.

A good starting point is a high-visibility cycling vest. Yes, it looks dorky, but it is likely to save your life. As I often tell my kids, I'd rather be a dorky-looking cyclist than a cool-looking corpse. Vests are also cheap. However, for real safety you also need good bike lights — even during the day. A bus driver once told me he loves it when cyclists use lights in the day, because then he can see them from two blocks away. Ever since then I always use lights, day or night. I have a complete guide to bike lights on my web site, with clickable lights to great lights — just go to http://averagejoecyclist.com/bike-lights-complete-guide/.

Your life is worth a $10 bike light — actually, it's worth the most expensive set of bike lights you could buy, and then some. If you're going to cheap out, cheap out on your cycling jersey, not your lights!

Many of the new electric bikes feature built-in light systems, wired to the main battery. Some of these even come on automatically when you cycle, like running lights on cars. Other new electric bikes feature dynamo lights connected to the wheels, which also come on as soon as you set off. These are great ideas. However, if you are considering such a bike, take a good, hard look at the lights. Some of them are adequate, but some will merely make you a bit more visible, while not enabling you to see very well at night. If that's the case but you still want the bike, spend some money on an extra set of lights. Your next-of-kins will thank you when they don't have to identify your body down at the morgue.

In order to shop for really good lights, it helps to know a bit about them, so I have included some information about bike lights.

Average Joe Cyclist Guide

Categories of Bike Lights

The first thing to know is that bike lights are designed for two main categories: lights to use on mountain bikes; and lights to use on the road while commuting. They have in common that they cost money and provide light, but they are very different in terms of weight, expense, how long they run and how much light they produce. So start off by deciding which type you need (read the sections below to decide).

How Bike Light Power is Measured

The Lumen has been adopted by most manufacturers as the unit for measuring brightness, now that Light Emitting Diodes (LEDs) are standard. So you can compare power based on lumens. Bear in mind however that while 900 lumens is ultra bright when focused in a laser-like beam, it becomes less bright when diffused into a wide angle beam. So you have to factor in beam width as well as power when assessing the efficacy of lights.

Road/Commuter Bike Lights

The good news is that road/commuter bike lights are cheaper than mountain bike lights. Their main point is to make you visible so that cars don't mow you down, and of course to enable you to see.

Important criteria to consider when choosing lights include:

- Power (measured in lumens)
- Beam (a powerful light that is dispersed too widely becomes less powerful)
- Battery life
- Side visibility
- Weight
- How easy they are to take on and take off (BEWARE lights that require you to take the whole thing off the bike to change the batteries.

This is common with cheap lights, and is a terrific nuisance)
- How easy it is to replace or recharge the battery: a good light will open up easily. The less good ones require you to find a screwdriver to snap them open, which can be really annoying and time-consuming.

Beam (how broadly and well the light is dispersed) impacts the power by spreading it wider. This is often a challenge on commuter lights: the light is often focused to a laser sharp spot so that motorists can see your flashing little white light coming for a mile or two. That's great. BUT you also need to be able to see clearly so that you don't hit a brick or break your neck on a pothole.

Many cyclists cope with this problem by having two front lights:

- a small, flashing, bright one so that others can see them; and
- a bigger, more diffused one that enables them to see the road ahead.

The smaller lights always come with different modes, and the flashing mode greatly extends battery life while attracting more attention, so it's a win-win. The wider lights that are designed for you to see where you are going often don't have a flashing mode, as this would just give you a headache (no one uses disco lights to navigate).

You can buy your bike lights separate or in sets (front and rear light together). You might get a better deal on a set, but the drawback is that sometimes one of the lights is less stellar than the other. As the savings are usually quite minor, I generally prefer to buy lights separately.

Here are some options to choose from. As there are hundreds to choose from, this is not meant to be an exhaustive list, just a representative sampling.

Average Joe Cyclist Guide

Front Lights for Road/Commuter Bikes

CatEye Econom HL-EL340 Front Light

CatEye is a brand known for quality, which is obviously what you want from something that could save your life. This front light is powerful enough so that you can ride reasonably fast, while not being too horrible for oncoming cyclists. A nice plus is the little side lights that improve side visibility. You can buy these from your lbs (local bike shop), as well as from Amazon for less than $50.

Niterider MiNewt.600

Reader and blogger Melanie Suzanne recommends the Niterider MiNewt 600 and says it is just as bright as car headlights:

> "My commute is along unlit ruralish/suburban streets and an unlit bike trail with lots of deer."

If it's good enough for that, it's probably good enough for most cyclists. It is USB rechargeable, so you can charge it while you work. *BikeRadar* sees this light as a bit bulky for use on a helmet, but nonetheless calls it a "versatile bargain," and Niterider, the manufacturer, claims:

> "This compact light features best in class lumens per dollar ratio, tool-less quick release mounting and a retina searing 600 lumens of light output. With this much power on tap, the Cordless not only blasts your way through the city street, but the trail as well. The reflector and lens are custom tuned for bike riding application delivering a superior beam pattern when compared to off the shelf optics."

This light will set you back around US$150.

Electron Terra 2

Well regarded and rated, the Electron Terra 2 offers a double light with great running time, for a reasonable price (around US$150). Each light pumps out 120 lumens, and they can be arranged wider apart than shown in the photo. They boast Sanyo li-ion batteries, yet the price is not ridiculous (unlike the NiteRider Pro 1200 reviewed below). You can set the double lights up so that one is a spot light or flashing light, and one is a wide beam. Features include low-battery indicator and enhanced side visibility. Claimed run time is up to 20 hours, with both head units on low, or 5 hours on high.

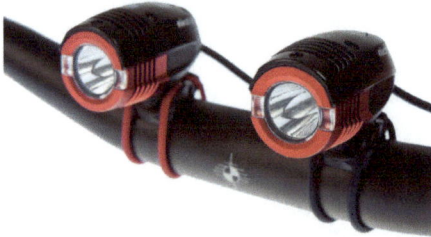

The Electron Terra 2 light is billed as a great light for a serious commuter, and even good enough for entry level night mountain bike riding. *Cycling Weekly* amusingly refers to it as a Wall-E lookalike. As a sci-fi enthusiast, I find this a plus!

Rear Lights for Road/Commuter Bikes

Cateye Rapid 3 (rear)

This rear light gives great visibility without completely blinding those behind you. A nice feature is that it switches back on in the mode in which you turned it off. This will be a relief to all those who get irritated at having to cycle through their light options every morning, trying to find the one and only mode that they use.

Run time is up to three hours on constant, 80 in flashing and 20 hours in rapid mode. It attaches via the new

Cateye FlexTight bracket, making mounting and taking it off easy. At less than $50, a great buy.

1W Portland Design Works Radbot 1000

Blogger Melanie Suzanne uses and recommends the 1W Portland Design Works Radbot 1000, which she calls the "Do Not Look Into Laser With Remaining Eye" light! Available from Amazon for a lot less than $50.

Mountain Bike Lights

These are all about the lighting power, so that you don't break your neck on a dark log on an unlit trail. Obviously you need more lighting power on a mountain trail than on a highway. Because mountain bikers need so much power, these lights are NOT cheap. Personally I will save my trail riding for the day time, but if you want to ride the trails at night and have the big bucks to finance it, here are some options.

Front Lights for Mountain Bikes

NiteRider Pro 1200 LED
Rechargeable HeadLight with Li-Ion Battery

I am throwing this one in because it's a respected make, but the price boggles my brain. It claims to be like having your own miniature sun, and to be the brightest bike lights ever constructed, producing 1,200 lumens via six of the highest performing Cree LEDs available. It is also complete customizable and comes with both helmet and bar mounts.

I battled to find customer reviews, and this is hardly surprising, because at the price (more than $500), I doubt that many people have bought them. I suspect that a lot of the cost comes from the Li-Ion battery, as these are never cheap.

The reviews I did find verified that the light is the brightest you can find, but also listed several complaints, including a couple that said the unit had failed right out of the box; several that said that the battery started to fade after an hour; many that complained that removing the battery to charge it was tricky; and most that complained that the set was too heavy (800 grams). I tend to agree with the reviewer who said that with this light, "NiteRider has lost the edge over their competition."

Light & Motion Seca 900 Ultra Bike Light

The Seca 900 Ultra Bike Light claims to be like a floodlight and to be one of the brightest bike lights ever made, and to have a long battery life. The hype includes "this high-powered light gives you the vision to ride just as fast on pitch-dark single track as you would on a mid-day downhill kamikaze run." Not sure why you'd want to do that, but if you do, it will cost you around $700.

Specs include a 9-cell Li-ion battery pack, a weight of 686 grams (240 oz), six Cree R2 LEDs (the highest rated LEDs available), and a claimed battery life of 3.5 hours on high and 7 hours on medium. Reviewers point out that it includes "a very high quality reflector to efficiently direct and sculpt the beam pattern to maximize light output;" the switches are easy to use; it exceeds the advertised 900 lumens; and at night on the trails it's like riding in a bubble of sunlight. The battery pack is big and unwieldy, but the consensus seems to be that this is the best light for your (big) bucks.

Rear Lights for Mountain Bikes

For obvious reasons, it is less necessary to be seen from the rear when you are cycling on a dark mountain than when you are whizzing down a dark highway. Therefore, any good rear light will do.

Other Cool Ways to be Seen on Your Bike

Reelight SL120 lights

Reelight SL120 lights (reviewed in detail on my blog) are a pair of front and back lights, powered by electrodynamic induction. This basically means that power is generated as your bike moves, by a pair of spoke-mounted magnets passing over a copper coil (inside the light unit). Once you have them mounted, they are always on. You don't have to remember to keep the batteries charged, or even to switch them on. As long as you're moving, your Reelight SL120 lights are on. There are just two downsides to Reelight SL120 lights: if you have disk brakes or a BionX bike, it can be tricky to line them up correctly; and the light they generate is minimal. Reelight SL120 lights are way better than nothing, but they are definitely insufficient on their own for night riding. They will not enable you to see the road ahead of you, and they are not bright enough (in my opinion) for you to be safe from cars.

Fun Lights! MonkeyLectric Lights

On a lighter note, some companies are coming up with excellent, fun ways for cyclists to be seen. For example, MonkeyLectric makes light sets that consist of 32 tiny, full-colour LED lights, mounted on a flat, kind-of-boot-shaped piece of plastic that fits perfectly onto the spokes of a bike wheel. It's dead easy to install – you basically tie it to the spokes with three plastic ties (included – unless you mess it up by putting it on backwards the first time, and have to cut one of the ties off, and then have to cycle, cursing and swearing, to the nearest hardware store to pick up another one – and who would be dumb enough to do that?). Then you put in three AA batteries, and you're good to go. Install time totals less than five minutes (time does not include cycling to the hardware store to get a new plastic tie).

Once mounted, the lights are controlled by four buttons, for Power, Speed, Color and Pattern. You can program in all sorts of fun patterns with this – for example, at Christmas time I program the lights to be green and red stars. I get a lot of smiles, as I look like a moving Christmas tree. As soon as you pick up speed, the rapidly whirling 32 lights generate very bright, highly visible, light patterns. The batteries last a really long time, too. Oh, and the set is very waterproof – I frequently cycle through monsoon-like downpours, and sometimes snow, and the lights are just fine.

These lights are just plain fun. This may sound weird, but when I'm setting off for work on a pitch dark morning in the rain, it cheers me up to have these bright lights whirling in my front wheel. I don't know why, but the lights make the dark and cold less depressing.

Also, my two sets of MonkeyLectric Lights make me extremely visible. I already had five lights on my bike, but the MonkeyLectric Lights have taken my visibility and shininess to a whole new level. Especially from the side. This is VERY useful in situations where an oncoming motorist is making a left-hand turn, and I have the right of way as I am going straight through the intersection. In these situations I have often had the experience that – despite my lights and high-visibility vest – the motorist just somehow does not see me. However, the MonkeyLectric Lights have made a dramatic difference. Motorists see me a LOT more quickly than previously, and screech to a halt much sooner – which makes for a much less terrifying experience for me. I seriously believe that at some point, these lights will actually save me from being hit, and perhaps even save my life.

Finally, it's kind of fun to have other cyclists (and a lot of little kids) really admire my cool lights! Once I cycled past a man and his son, and I clearly heard the little boy say:

"I want a bike like that one!"

It's nice to be a role mode! Bottom line: I highly

recommend these lights to anyone who rides in the dark, and wants to have fun and be safe while they're doing it. Other companies are also coming up with lights that can be fitted to the rims of bike wheels, and it's all good.

Bicycle Bells

It's also really important for cyclists to be heard. The $5 you spend on a bicycle bell may be the best $5 you ever spend. It's an excellent, polite way to let pedestrians and other cyclists know that you are about to go past them (and as an electric biker, you will constantly be overtaking other cyclists). On a couple of occasions I have used my bell to alert people about someone else's bike, and averted a collision on their behalf. Unfortunately, someone somewhere seems to have decreed that bicycle bells are not cool. To which I say two things:

- They were cool enough for Queen, and no one can say they weren't cool!
- I'd rather be alive and uncool than dead and cool.

Basic Tools to
Carry with You

L ike other cyclist-commuters, electric bike commuters should try to carry a set of basic bike tools with them: a spare tube and tire levers; some small hex wrenches (Allen keys); a patch kit; a straight blade screwdriver; and a small adjustable wrench.

OR you can just carry a credit card, and call a cab if you ever get stuck. I recommend this alternative for people who are not so good at the techie side of cycling. If you're going to use this method, make sure you get your bike serviced regularly, and use puncture-resistant tires. The few bucks you spend on services and good tires will be a lot less than what you could end up spending on cabs!

That said, many of the new electric bikes aim to be as close to maintenance-free as possible. The new internal hubs mean your gear sprockets are not exposed to the elements, and so are much less likely to get dirty, wet and break down. Some electric bikes even have internal wiring for lights and other cables. I love this idea, and aim to one day own a maintenance-free bike where all the parts that can break or need to be oiled are completely hidden away. These bikes are also good for those who like to cycle in smart clothes, as there is no chance of getting bike grease on your clothing.

Generally speaking, the less techie you are, the more useful it would be to have a low-maintenance bike. Kind of a no-brainer, but worth saying, nonetheless.

Types of Electric Bikes

Although there are an almost dizzying amount of different electric bikes, there are a limited number of types of electric bikes. You can begin your search by narrowing down what type of electric bike you want. This will depend entirely on your priorities, that is, on what you really want to do with your bike. Perhaps you are clear that you merely want to commute with your electric bike. Or perhaps you want an electric bike purely for recreation, maybe to go exploring when you are on an RV trip. Once you are clear on your priorities, it will be easier to choose between the following types of electric bikes.

Electric Hybrid Bikes

Hybrid bikes are a great choice for all-round versatility. As their name implies, they are a blend of traditional road bikes (which are built for speed) and mountain bikes (which are built to be tough). As a result, they're tougher than road bikes, but not as heavy as mountain bikes. Some have suspension; some do not. They are a good choice if you want to commute, or if you want to ride the local trails. These bikes really are ideal for commuting purposes, as they are strong enough to withstand potholes and carry your luggage. However, they are not as heavy as mountain bikes, so you do not have to deal with unnecessary extra weight.

Electric Mountain Bikes

You could commute on a mountain bike, but it would be slower than commuting on a hybrid bike. But as they are tougher, you would be able to jump on and off curbs!

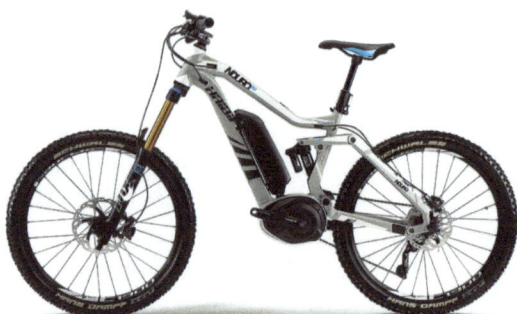

On the other hand, if your primary goal is to explore trails or to bike on mountains, then you need a mountain bike. A front suspension mountain bike will probably do you just fine. If however you are fearless and athletic, you might want to consider a full-suspension mountain bike, such as the beautiful Haibike above, so that you can hurtle down mountains, leap over logs, grab some "big air" and just generally carry on like a weekend warrior. With the aid of your electric motor, you could be mistaken for a pro rider!

Like all mountain bikes, an electric mountain bike needs to be able to deal with obstacles such as rocks and logs. However, with electric mountain bikes there are special considerations. First, the electric components need to be tough enough to deal with the rough conditions. Because of a higher likelihood of exposure to water, the cables and their connections need to be properly sealed.

Either a crank drive or a chain drive motor will do, but the bike should have gears, as you will certainly be climbing up hills (they basically come with the territory if you want to bike on a mountain). At this point in time crank drive motors are less common; however many believe that they are the best suited for mountain bikes as there is less friction, they are sealed better, and in general they perform better on hills. It is likely that in the future we will see more electric mountain bikes with crank drive engines.

In terms of power, an electric mountain bike should be on the higher end, preferably between 500 watts and 750 watts, to cope with the demands of steep hills. Note that various jurisdictions have different laws for maximum size of bike engine, and that in some places the law is different for on-road and off-road usage. Generally speaking, your local dealer will not be selling motors that are illegal in your area.

In planning your purchase and your trips, bear in mind that the advertised mileage on batteries is achieved under laboratory conditions – and on a mountain, you will definitely not be under laboratory conditions! So work on the assumption that your range will be only half what was advertised, to avoid getting stuck with a heavy bike and a flat battery on top of a remote mountain.

Brakes are a special consideration for electric mountain bikes. Often mountain bikes are equipped with V-brakes, and these are just fine for regular mountain bikes. However with an electric assist – especially a 500 to 750 watt motor – you are going to be moving a whole lot faster, and V-brakes will not suffice. You will be moving like a pro cyclist, and you will need the same kind of stopping power they depend on. This means that disc brakes on your electric mountain bike are essential. They offer improved stopping power in general, and especially under rough conditions. Moreover, they require relatively little maintenance, for which you will be grateful when you return exhausted from conquering a mountain, with a very muddy bike!

Another aspect that is important with electric mountain bikes is shock absorption. This is important for all mountain bikes, and the intensity of your riding style will dictate whether you go for front shock absorption only, or whether you get dual suspension (also called full suspension). Bear in mind that the shocks will not only be protecting you – they will also be protecting the engine, battery and other electrical components. Which means the better your shock absorption, the longer your system will last. On the other hand, dual suspension is not really a great idea for electric bikes, as the suspended rear section can wobble sideways, making the bike unstable at the kind of high speeds you can achieve on an electric bike.

The frame, tires and wheels should be very strong, to stand up to the combination of rough terrain and speed.

Optibikes are an example of electric mountain bikes. They are very expensive, but reputedly very good.

Electric City Bikes (Cruisers, Comfort, Urban Bikes)

These are usually steel bikes, with fatter tires than usual. They are not as efficient as most other bikes, but they are fun. Some of the newer ones combine modern components with creative retro styling. They usually have a comfortable, upright sitting position. They are intended to be used for cruising in style to the coffee shop, perhaps running a few errands, and then meeting up with friends. In short, these are bikes for short, leisure-oriented trips. The assumption is that there will be few, if any, hills, and that neither speed nor carrying heavy cargoes are high priorities.

These bikes are perfect for adaptation as electric bikes, as they are designed for a casual, sweat-free cycling experience, and an electric assist makes that much more achievable for a wider range of people.

While speed is not important for city bikes, torque and acceleration are important. This is because the nature of trips in the city is to have frequent stops; therefore to make sure the experience is as easy and sweat-free as possible, it is useful for the bikes to have good acceleration capabilities. Also, as stop-start travelling drains batteries rapidly, the bikes need to have good batteries.

Throttles are useful for this type of travelling, as they make pulling off quickly from red lights much easier.

Folding Electric Bikes

Folding bikes typically are smaller and lighter than regular bikes, with shorter wheelbases and smaller wheels. The seating position is very upright, making them ideal for cycling in traffic. Folding bikes are a good choice for combination transit options – such as biking to the station, taking the train, then biking from the train station to work – and then sliding the bike tidily under your desk for the day! They are also good for short distance commutes, as you can just fold them up and take them into wherever you are going. (With regular bikes, the hassle of locking them up sometimes means that for very short commutes, walking is easier.)

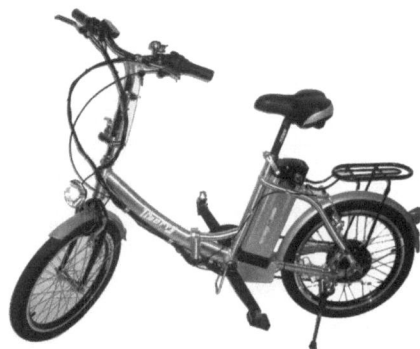

Folding bikes are designed to be light, so that people can easily carry them around. Of course, the catch with folding electric bikes is that the motor inevitably adds weight to the bike. While an average folding bike might weigh between 20 and 30 pounds, adding a motor typically takes it up to between 40 and 50 pounds. For some commuters, a 40-pound bike can be just too heavy to carry. Fortunately, some of them can be rolled along.

When buying an electric folding bike, it's important to make sure that the folding mechanism is not hampered by the engine. This is unlikely to be the case with folding bikes that are designed to have engines, but may be a problem when the folding bike is retrofitted with an engine – particularly if you do it yourself. In any event, check this carefully before buying. Ideally you want a folding electric bike that folds easily and correctly, that is light enough for you to carry short distances, and that can be easily rolled along when it is folded. This would give you enormous travelling flexibility.

Another thing to consider if buying a folding electric

bike is whether the bike has gears. Some do, some do not, and this could be a problem if you plan to cycle up any hills. Also, some folding electric bikes come with suspension, and this could really save you some discomfort if you are using your bike in a city. I always find it amusing that mountain bikes were designed to smooth out bumps in the countryside, but trails are often a lot smoother than downtown city roads. I regularly hurt myself on unexpected potholes in urban areas, and once, in the dark, hit a pothole so deep that I broke the rim of my hybrid bike and injured my back. And this was on a designated bike route!

If you want a folding bike, some dealers sell a selection of the top-class Brompton folding bike, complete with pre-installed BionX systems. One of the best such stores is NYCeWheels in New York, an extremely reputable company with in-depth expertise in electric bikes – check them out if you are anywhere near New York.

Tricycles

Tricycles are three-wheeled bikes that offer increased stability. They may be used by those who have physical challenges of various sorts. For example, they are a great option for seniors who wish to rediscover biking, but are afraid of falling. Many manufacturers offer electric trikes.

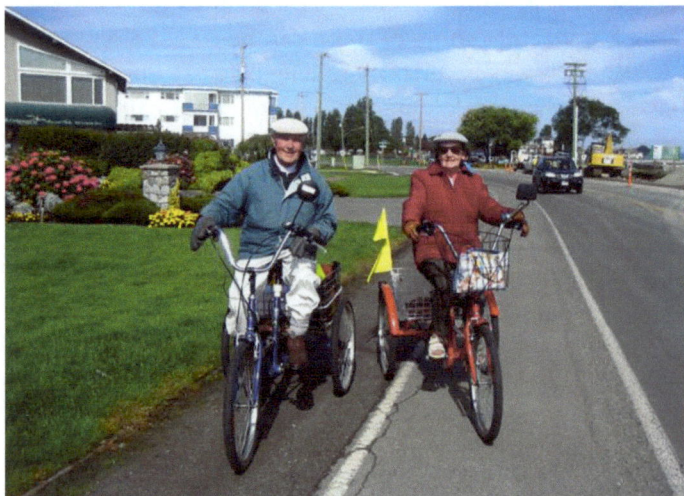

Average Joe Cyclist Guide

Types of Electric Motors for Bikes

Brushed and Brushless Motors

Motors for electric bikes may be brushed, or they may be brushless DC motors (BLDC motors). The industry default has become brushless motors, because generally they are quieter, smaller, and lighter. However, there are some knowledgeable people in the industry who support brushed motors, maintaining that they are more robust and reliable, that they are a relatively cheap way (in terms of cost and power) to gain hill-climbing ability, and that they are cheap and simple to service and don't have to be serviced often.

The average user does not have to think about this issue, as most electric bikes are sold with brushless motors, due to the fact that they are more efficient at producing power, and therefore the battery lasts longer.

Sensorless or Permanent Magnet BLDC Motors

This is a new innovation, and promises to make BLDC (brushless DC) motors more reliable. These motors do not require sensors as the position of the armature is detected using magnetic field detection. This reduces the notoriously large amount of electronics required on the motor, resulting in higher reliability.

Again, this is an issue that the average user does not have to think about. If sensorless BLDC motors live up to their early promise, they will simply become the industry norm, and will be the default engine on whatever bike you are considering.

Crank Drive Motors

Crank drive motors were the first advanced electric bike motors, and were developed in Japan in the early 1990s by Panasonic and Yamaha. As the name clearly indicates, they are situated in the crank (the crank set being the round thing that cleverly converts the energy from your legs into energy that moves the chain and therefore moves the bike). These motors drive additional power (over and above your own leg power) through the rear gear system.

Crank drive motors can be adjusted to suit different environments, and are widely thought to be the best motors because they allow you to use the bikes gears to get up hills, or to haul heavy loads. That said, I get up enormous hills with my 350-watt hub drive electric bike. Nonetheless, the general wisdom is that if you know you are going to have to climb very steep hills (more than 17%), you are better off with a crank drive motor.

Hub Motors

As the early crank drive motors were so expensive, hub motors were developed as a cheaper alternative. These motors, again as the name indicates, are mounted in the

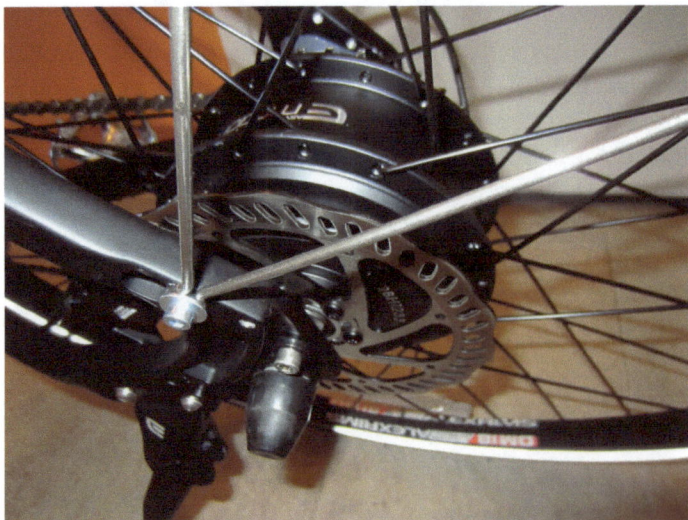

hub (the center part) of the wheel, usually the rear wheel. These are now the most common motors. They basically have only one gear, so although some of them are very powerful, they are not ideal for hilly areas. If you live in a flat city, these are just fine.

That said, many of the large hub drive motors have amazing hill capacity. For example, the high torque BionX motors cope very well with hills: I can vouch for the fact that the latest BionX high-end, high-power systems take you up hills as if you truly are bionic. Actually they exert so much torque that I managed to break a bike frame. However, that is rare, and it must be admitted that it happened when I was still pretty chubby … huge hills, chubby guy, maximum torque … you do the math.

Friction Drive Motors

These are simple, light motors, that basically work by spinning a roller that is pressed against the bicycle's tire. There is a limit to how much power can be put through a friction drive, because the acceleration is dependent on the roller maintaining solid contact with a small patch of the tire.

These engines have their proponents, but they are very much in the minority. I would say that friction motors are better suited to techie people who like to assemble engines themselves, using parts from model airplanes.

Note that with these systems, the roller and/or the tire usually wear out after just a few hundred miles. So although they may seem cheap, they won't last long, which means they are not usually cheap.

So my advice is to avoid friction motors – unless you plan to scarcely use the bike at all (and if this was the case, you probably would not be taking the trouble to read this).

What Size Motor
Should You Buy?

As with every other question about your new electric bike, the answer to this one comes down to personal needs and choice. Will your daily commute take you off road, and over the top of a mountain? If so, you are going to need the kind of big, tough motor that is found on, for example, Optibikes. Their top of the line mountain bike is powered by a **48 V** lithium ion battery with Cool CarbonTM 1100 watts Motorized Bottom BracketTM. With this, you could commute over mountains without much trouble. On the other hand, if your commute is more conservative, your needs will be similarly less conservative.

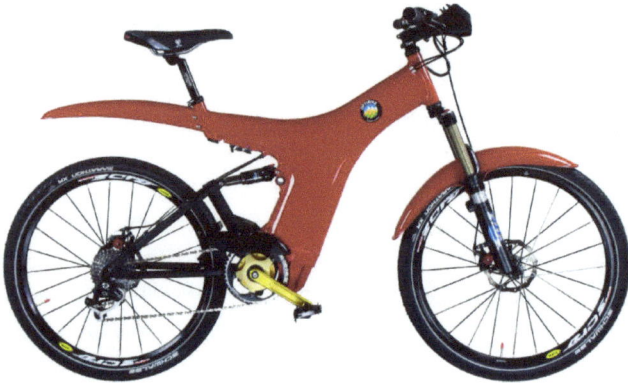

Like Optibikes, BionX offers a whole range of motor sizes, so you can choose something that meets your needs. Examining the range of sizes on their web site will give you an idea of the options out there (www.bionx.ca). Their Premium series pairs their SL 350 HT DT XL* motor with an extra long-range **48 V** battery, and claims a range of 105 km (65 mi.). This is a **350 watts** (W) motor. At the other end of the range, their PL 250 M is a much smaller motor, at 250 W. However, I used one of these for years, and it easily sufficed for my needs. At the time, I was not doing any hills, and just needed a boost so that my long commute would be faster and less daunting. I upgraded to one of their 350 W motors when my commute changed to include a couple of steep hills. (Bear in mind that I weighed just under 200 pounds for most of this time.)

In a nutshell, you should not be looking at a motor smaller than 250 W if you have to deal with hills. And if you weigh more than 200 pounds, your minimum should be 350 W. Unless you are riding a bike such as my Emotion Race Bike, which cleverly combines gear power with a crank-drive 250 W motor. With this bike, I can climb major hills without too much sweat.

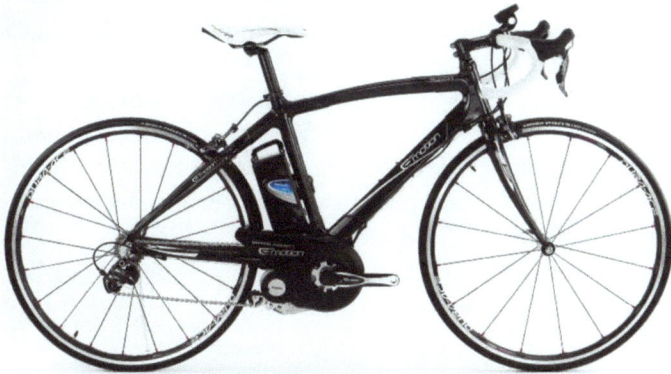

A 350 W motor will meet most needs, and will take a heavy cyclist up big hills with minimal sweat (but **not** without pedaling). After that, the bigger the motor, the more power you have. The 500 W motor is very powerful. The 750 W motor is tremendously powerful. The 1100 W offered by Optibikes is insanely powerful, but the price tag matches the power.

But bear in mind that the bigger the motor, the bigger the battery you need. So a powerful 500 W engine will need a big battery, making for a heavy combination.

Also, bear in mind that none of these sizes gives you a motor scooter. All the way up to 750 W, you still have to do some pedaling. But that's a good thing. If you didn't want to pedal and get fit, presumably you'd be reading a book about motorcycles.

Finally, keep in mind that there are laws about the size of motor that electric bikes can have. In the EU, Japan, China, and other countries, the power limit is 250 watts. In Canada, 350-watt engines are common. Eight of Canada's provinces allow electric power assisted bicycles, and in seven of these, they are limited to 500 watts output. In the province of Alberta the limit is 750 watts. In the USA, the limit is 750 watts. In the UK cyclists are severely limited, and the motor's maximum continuous rated power output must not exceed 200 W for bicycles, 250 W for bicycle tandems (i.e. two seaters) and 250 W for tricycles. I am completely confident that this will change as the reality of gas shortages finally dawns on the United Kingdom's legislators.

Usually you will not be able to buy motors that are too big for the laws of your own country (although with internet orders, it is possible to get around this). Also, highly technical people can put together motors that exceed legislative limits. For the average buyer, it will suffice to be guided by the advice and knowledge of a reputable dealer.

Other Issues to Consider when Buying

Price

The price will be one of the first things most buyers will consider. How much you can afford comes down to how much money you have; how badly you want it; and how much money you plan to save by using your electric bike instead of your car. I usually focus on the last point when trying to persuade my wife that we need a new electric bike. Joking aside, your electric bike definitely will save you money if you use it instead of a car.

Calculating how much it will save is complex and personal, as it depends for example on whether you drive a Porsche 911 or a Fiat 500. Then there is also the fact that the electric bike will make a positive contribution to your health, whereas driving a car is known to accelerate the ageing process, due to the stress attached. In fact, if you do one of those quizzes where they assess your actual age as opposed to your biological age, one of the questions they ask is how many hours a day do you spend driving. The more hours you routinely spend driving, the older you really are. This fact in itself would be enough to make me give up my car, if I still had one.

Apart from weighing up your personal needs and finances, bear in mind that when electric bikes are very cheap, there is a simple reason: they are usually very poor quality. The old adage of you get what you pay for is very apt when it comes to buying bikes, whether electric or not. Most of the electric bikes in the world are in China, and the rest of the world is currently being flooded with cheap electric bikes from China. I am not saying that every bike that comes out of China is garbage – but I am saying do not be blinded by a low price. You take your life in your hands whenever you go on a public road, whether in a car or on a bike. Personally I will not trust my life to a cheaply-made vehicle of any sort.

Range

The range of the bike is, of course, how far you can ride on one charge. The problem is how to assess this. All electric bikes will be advertised as having a particular range. However, these advertised ranges are usually not accurate. In fact, sometimes they are downright exaggerated, and may even be four times higher than the reality.

Also if you think about it, it is impossible for range claims to be totally accurate. There are too many factors that make it different from person to person. These include how much the rider weighs; how much assistance the rider chooses; the terrain they're cycling over; the amount of luggage they're carrying; how hard they're pedaling; wind conditions; what kind of battery they're using; and how fast they're going. For example, if you decide to engage no assistance at all because you're on flat terrain and you're feeling strong, your range is as far as you can go before you collapse – which for some people might be 200 miles, and for others could be 20. On the other hand, if you engage the highest level of assistance constantly, and are in very hilly terrain, you can eat through your battery power pretty fast. But if you have a lithium battery, you're going to keep going a lot longer than if you have a nickel-cadmium battery, as lithium batteries have a higher energy density (see below, "What Kind of Battery should you Buy?")

As a starting point, it's safe to assume that the range is lower than what the manufacturer says it is. Advertised ranges are based on laboratory conditions, and you are not going to be cycling in a laboratory. Moreover, the manufacturer is free to make up whatever range they like, as there is no International Standard for calculating electric bike ranges, such as exists in the USA for calculating EPA (Environmental Protection Agency) car mileage ratings. And even real world car mileages don't match up to the EPA ratings, even though they are stringently controlled. This is because there are so many variables around the way real people drive real cars in the real world that it's ridiculous to think we could achieve a completely accurate rating of average miles per gallon. And when it comes to bikes there isn't even a standard to which manufacturers are held, so it's pretty much still the Wild West when it comes to range claims.

So all you can do is find out as much as possible. If you are buying from a reputable, knowledgeable electric bike dealer (and you should be), ask the dealer how the range was calculated, and under what conditions it was calculated (such as what speed was used, and how much the rider was pedaling). You can also ask the dealer if they have tested the bike themselves and managed to achieve the advertised range.

As with all products, the claims are likely to be more accurate if you are buying from a reputable dealer. And as with all bike-related products, quality tends to come with a price tag. If the bike is very cheap, the performance and the range are sure to reflect that.

The bottom line is that the range claimed is very much a paper claim – which is not to say that it is certain to be wildly inaccurate, but just to say that you should not take it on blind faith. It's also very helpful to spend some time Googling the bike you have in mind, and see what real world users have to say.

Throttle vs. Pedal Assist

There are basically two ways in which electric bikes assist you:

1. Some have a throttle, which allows you to activate the power assist with a simple flick of your thumb. Usually these have hub motors. The throttle usually allows you to move the bike without pedaling at all (although this would rapidly deplete most batteries, so it is not advisable except in an emergency situation).
2. Others have a pedal assist, in which the amount of assist is proportional to the amount of pedaling.

That said, there are also electric bikes that combine

both types of assist – BionX kits, for example. When I use my BionX bike, I usually use only the pedal assist, but I do employ the throttle on a hill start, or when I suddenly have an irrational urge to overtake someone, or when a hill is particularly, annoyingly steep. In my opinion, bikes that allow you to coast along without even pedaling kind of defeat the purpose of getting fit. However, for people with serious physical limitations, this can be a very good thing. And also, a throttle combined with a hub motor can come in very handy:

BionX to the Rescue – in the Snow!

One winter morning I woke up before dawn and decided to get to work before the traffic picked up. The night before the weather forecast had promised clear skies, so I set off at my usual rapid pace on my trusty BionX commuter bike.

About two miles into the ride it started to rain. Expletive! Well, I had a rain-resistant jacket on, so I wasn't too concerned. As I pedaled on, it dawned on me that the rain was unusually cold. Downright freezing, in fact. Finally my still-sleepy brain put it together: rain + freezing = freezing rain! Double expletive! After a moment or two of hesitation I decided to push on up the hill – perhaps it was just a fleeting shower. I continued on up, feeling as if the North Pole was screaming into my face.

By the time I neared the top of the hill, the silence of snow had descended all around me. Pedestrians were wandering across the quiet street ahead of me, confident that no cars were around because it was so silent. My bell was too frozen to work, so I resorted to yelling: "Bike coming through!" Even going uphill, my BionX electric bike is pretty fast, and I did not want to mow anyone down. The pedestrians turned to stare at me in shock. I could just see them thinking, "Look at that crazy person cycling in the snow." As I went by them, I yelled out "The weather forecast said it was going to be clear!" (while doing my best to stay upright and look entirely sane).

I was halfway to work, so there seemed to be no choice but to press on. Besides, my bike was handling the snow pretty well. I suspect the extra weight of the BionX electric motor kit helped to keep me firmly upright.

Unfortunately, I was not dressed for snow. Parts of me were getting soaked to the skin, and I knew I had to get to work before hypothermia set in. But then disaster struck. Under the onslaught of being freezing cold and soaked in snow, my drive chain stopped working. I was trying to pedal, but the gears just kept slipping.

Of course, that was when my trusty BionX electric engine kicked in! Undeterred by the elements, it continued to work smoothly, and I cruised sedately all the way to work, even though I could hardly pedal at all.

Finally I squelched in, parked the dripping bike, and had the best hot shower of my life! The only negative thing was that I was so early that there was no one to see me arrive, covered from head to foot in snow. I was feeling pretty darn proud of myself for making it to work despite the snow, but sadly there was no one to admire me.

To Regenerate or Not?

Some electric bikes incorporate a regenerative aspect, that is, they can recharge the battery as you go downhill, and also when you engage the brakes, if you put them in negative assist mode. This is billed as a bonus feature, and it might work for you. Definitely it does have the advantage of saving wear and tear on your brakes. However, those who don't use them, such as Elite Electric Bikes, claim:

"Our bicycles don't have a battery recharge capability because we use geared motors. We believe that the extra weight and cost of the recharging components are not worth it for the 5% extra charging benefit that you might get from pedal recharging. Plus a geared motor allows the bike to freewheel with no drag like on regenerative models, so if you run out of juice, you can pedal without resistance."

The last claim is not really valid – on most bikes that can regenerate, if you switch off the motor (or the battery runs out of power), there is zero drag and you are free to freewheel to your heart's content.

However, personally, I find that the amount of energy my BionX bike generates on downhills is minimal, and also that the system that makes it work can actually be a hassle. In fact, I think the regenerative braking system is the only negative feature on the otherwise excellent BionX system. It's a little bit fussy, and can sometimes result in having no power at all, because the trigger mechanism is out by about the width of a mouse's cornea, and this throws out the whole electric circuit. Once you know what's causing it, you can adjust on the fly – but the first time it happened to me, I was stranded. Plus, I find it annoying to suddenly lose power. It is possible to bypass the system, but this does not work very well, in my experience.

Bottom line, in my opinion, is that it's an unnecessary and complicated frill – and besides, most electric bikes don't have them. BionX is one of the few that do.

What if the Battery Runs out?

Elite Bikes claims:

"Our bikes are much lighter 23 to 25 kg (50 to 55 pounds) than scooters or older/cheaper electric bikes. They also use a geared motor instead of a direct drive motor, which means that there is no motor drag when the bike is used without electric assist. For both of these reasons, you can ride our bikes just like a normal bike if the battery runs out before you arrive at your destination. Our bikes have a battery charge indicator so you can monitor your battery power to avoid this situation."

Well, the reality is that whether the motor is geared or direct drive, you CAN ride it if the battery runs out. This is one of the great things about electric bikes: they are bikes, not scooters or cars, and so if the engine stops working, you can still get around on them. You are highly unlikely to be stranded, even with zero battery power.

What Kind of Battery Should You Buy?

Often this is not a question you need to ask, as it will follow from your choice of bike and engine. There is likely to be a battery that comes with your bike, so you won't have to think about it. And of course if you are buying a very large motor, then you should also be getting a very large battery. If you are buying from a reputable dealer, this will all be taken care of.

However, in many cases you will have to think about battery choices, so it's best to have enough knowledge to make a wise choice. Also, bear in mind that there are an amazing number of manufacturers who claim that their batteries offer the greatest range, period. Logically they cannot all be correct, so it follows that you need to take manufacturers' claims with a large pinch of salt, and be knowledgeable enough to know a little bit about what you are buying. First, it is necessary to understand a bit about battery terminology.

How Battery Power is Measured

Volts, Amps and Watts

Power is measured in Watts. This measurement applies to the bike's motor. To determine the Watts, multiply as follows:

- Voltage (volts) x Current (amps) = Power (watts).

Further, volts and amps are defined as follows:
- **Volts**: potential to do work. Think of volts like the pressure of water in a closed hosepipe. The potential is there, but potential on its own does nothing.
- **Amps**: these may be thought of as the current that unleashes the volt potential, turning it into power (hence, volts x amps = watts). Using the hosepipe

analogy again, the amps can be thought of as the current of water flowing through the hose.

Battery capacity is usually measured in Watt-hrs

Watt-hrs = amp-hrs x volts (that is, power is equivalent to how long the current will be applied to the battery's potential, multiplied by the amount of potential the battery has)

Note: battery capacity may also be given in amp-hrs, but this is insufficient, as it does not include the voltage, so it does not reflect the true energy capacity. So if a bike is advertised with a 1000 watt motor and has a 36 volt battery, with a capacity of 9 amp hrs, then the true capacity of the battery is 9 x 36, that is, 324 watt hrs (written as 324 Wh).

Watt-hrs is important, because watt-hrs determine the range of your bike, that is, how far you can go. (See also "Range" above.)

Bearing all of the above in mind will help you to evaluate manufacturers' advertisements and claims for their batteries. In general, you want a battery with a minimum of 200 watt-hrs.

Types of Batteries

Lead-acid Batteries (SLA)

Lead-acid batteries are cheap and easy to recycle. However, they are sensitive to bad treatment, and they don't last very long. They are not a good choice if you're serious about actually using your bike to commute.

Lead-acid batteries are cheap for several good reasons: they weigh twice as much as NiMh batteries, and three times as much as lithium batteries. They have much less usable capacity than NiMh batteries or lithium batteries. They only last for half as long as nickel or lithium batteries.

Warning: if a cheap electric bike is advertised and the advert does not state what kind of battery it has, you can pretty much be certain that it has a lead-acid battery. It might be cheap, but it's not a bargain. It might be good enough if you want the bike as a mere toy, to be taken out and played with occasionally in your immediate neighborhood – but if not, it would be better to avoid these batteries altogether.

Nickel-cadmium (NiCd) Batteries

Weight for weight, nickel-cadmium (NiCd) batteries have more capacity than lead-acid battery, and capacity is an important consideration on a bike. However, nickel-cadmium is expensive and cadmium is a nasty pollutant and hard to recycle. On the other hand, NiCd batteries will last longer than lead-acid batteries. But the reality is that because they are so hard to recycle or get rid of safely, NiCd batteries are rapidly becoming a thing of the past. These are also not a good choice, regardless of price.

Nickel–metal Hydride (NiMh) Batteries

NiMh batteries are somewhat more efficient than NiCd batteries, but they are also more expensive. Most people's report that NiMh offers little improvement in range over NiCd. On the other hand, they will last longer and are easier to dispose of correctly. Nonetheless, NiMH batteries are also becoming a rarity, because the market place is being taken over by Lithium-ion (Li-ion) batteries.

Lithium-ion (Li-ion) Batteries

These have become the default battery, capturing over 90% of the market. To complicate matters, there are many different kinds of Li-ion batteries. On the plus side, Li-ion batteries last longer and generate more power for their weight than other batteries. On the negative side, they are fussy little creatures, and require a genius-inspired smorgasbord of electronic features to prevent them from self-destruction and even catching fire! Of course, none of those are your problems, as the manufacturer will have sorted out the genius side. But like all good things in life, this comes at a price: the batteries are really very expensive, and show little sign of getting cheaper. For example, faced with the decision of buying a new Li-ion battery for my current BionX bike setup, I am seriously considering watching the sales and getting a whole new bike, considering the battery costs into the four figures!

I could of course find a cheaper one, but it would not last long, and also I really don't want my bike to catch fire. Alternatively, there are high tech suppliers who can recharge your old BionX battery for a reasonable price. There are even people who can figure out a way for you to use a cheaper, non-propriety brand of battery. In my experience none of these are as good or as safe as the genuine article, but they can be a lot cheaper.

Lithium-ion Polymer (Li-pol) Batteries

This is a new one, and promises to be no better than the Li-ion in terms of range, weight or price. However, it can be molded into interesting shapes. They contain no liquid, so they don't require the heavy protective cases that other batteries need. Also, this absence of free liquid theoretically means that they should be more stable and less vulnerable to problems caused by overcharge, damage or abuse. In general, they seem to be ideal for use in high capacity low power applications – such as electric bikes.

Given the new trend to make electric bikes look just like other bikes, I am guessing that some creative manufacturers will come up with some radically cool ideas. I wouldn't rush into buying one of these, however, until they prove themselves in terms of battery life.

Lithium Cobalt (LCO) Batteries

This is another variation on Li-ion. It's a relatively new kid on the block, and its proponents claim it has much higher energy density than other lithium batteries, so that it offers optimum power in a light, compact package. For example it is used in Optibikes, and the manufacturers claim "no other electric bike can go as far as an Optibike, guaranteed". Yet another one that still has to prove itself, though.

Lithium Manganese (LiMg204) Battery

This is another new kid on the block, and is the same battery technology used in the Nissan Leaf hybrid car. Some claim it is the best of all. For example it is used in Elite Electric Bikes, and the manufacturers claim that it lasts longer and generates more power than other Lithium batteries.

Wrapping up the Battery Debate

As you can see, it is hard to know whose claims to believe. It does seem however that lithium cobalt offers higher energy density, but that lithium manganese batteries are somewhat safer, and are more environmentally friendly. This comes from an unbiased source:

"Lithium Manganese provides a higher cell voltage than Cobalt based chemistries at 3.8 to 4 Volts but the energy density is about 20% less. It also provides additional benefits to Lithium-ion chemistry, including lower cost and higher temperature performance. This chemistry is more stable than Lithium Cobalt technology and thus inherently safer but the trade off is lower potential energy densities. Lithium Manganese cells are also widely available but they are not yet as common as Lithium Cobalt cells. Manganese, unlike Cobalt, is a safe and more environmentally benign cathode material. Manganese is also much cheaper than Cobalt, and is more abundant" (http://www.mpoweruk.com/lithiumS.htm)

In sum, the best choice is some kind of lithium ion battery, but the jury is still out on which is the best lithium battery. If the bike you are considering comes with any kind of lithium battery, you are off to a good start. Beyond that, you need to weigh up what is more important to you: proven safety and range (Li-ion); higher energy density (LCO); performance coupled with safety, but relatively new (LiMg204); cool shapes and cutting edge (Li-pol).

What Size Battery Should You Buy?

As a general rule of thumb, look for a setup in which the battery capacity in watt hrs is equal to the motor capacity in watts. This kind of setup will have the greatest range because the motor will not be over-taxing the battery. You should be able to get one hour at maximum assist with this setup.

As an example, the top-of-the-range BionX PL 350 HT DT L has a battery with 355 Wh. So the motor capacity and battery capacity in watt hrs is almost identical, and the battery is advertised as having an impressive range of 56 miles (90 km). Obviously it would take longer than an hour to cover 56 miles on an electric bike. This rating obviously factors in that some pedaling will be done, and that maximum assistance will not be continuously used. I have a similar setup, and I can vouch for the fact that maximum assistance at all times would be superfluous. Most people will only need maximum assistance on steep uphills.

Other Issues to Consider When Buying a Battery

How Long will the Battery Last Before it Needs Replacing?

This will depend on how hard you use it. The more you pedal on each trip, the longer your battery will last. Also, the dealer or manufacturer should be able to give you an idea of how long it will last. It's also not a bad idea to Google reviews of the battery, so as to find out what other users have experienced.

This is an important issue to keep in mind. If you are buying a good quality setup, buying a new battery will be a significant cost. If I were to start all over again with electric bikes, I would always buy two batteries up front. After all, I am eventually going to have to buy the second battery, and by buying it in the beginning, I get the convenience of having two batteries, so that I can extend my range when I need to. And because there are two of them, they should last as long as they would if I bought them back-to-back.

Can the Battery be Safely Disposed of?

Find out if it is recyclable, and if the dealer will recycle it for you. There are a lot of variations in this regard: some of the older style batteries are notoriously unfriendly to the environment. However, the evolving technology is taking this into account, and electric bike batteries are rapidly improving their environmental friendliness.

What about Other Battery Features?

Some batteries come with a USB port that you can use to charge or run your other devices, such as lights – a very handy feature, which gives you the potential to keep yourself safe with super bright lights. Most batteries come with a lock that is operated by a key, making it harder for thieves to remove it from your bike. More and more of them are being designed to provide power for the rear and front lights. This is an excellent feature that can make your life simpler. I don't have it yet, and I spend a lot of time making sure that all of my batteries are charged: bike battery, light batteries, etc.

Tip for Maintaining Your Battery

Once you have bought an expensive battery, don't let it die on you before its time. In particular, lithium batteries can die if left uncharged for too long. If you're not going to ride for more than a month (such as during winter), spend about $25 on a 7-day timer plug so that the battery can be automatically topped up for a short period (half an hour will do) once a week. This keeps the battery "exercised" and should prevent it from dying on you. Even if it does die on you (this happened to me once), a good techie shop can often nurse it back to life.

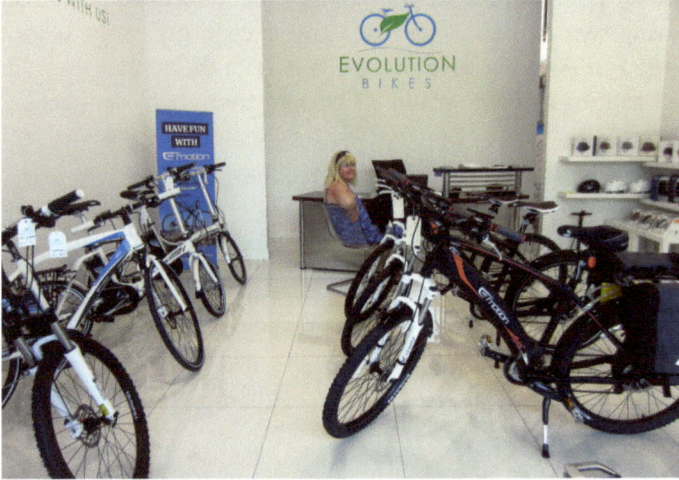

Think long and hard and consider all your options when buying your electric bike and your battery –
they are major investments. This photo shows Maggie (Mrs. Average Joe Cyclist) at Evolution Bikes on Vancouver's North Shore. This is an excellent bike shop with a very knowledgeable owner. We have bought several bikes there.

Practical Questions to Ask Before You Buy Your Electric Bike

Once you're ready to start shopping, pause for a moment to review your priorities. You should already have decided if you want a mountain bike, a commuter, a cruiser or a folding bike. Now consider the following issues:

- Will you need to travel long distances?
- Will you have to climb a lot of hills?
- Do you want to pedal all the time, or would you prefer the option of sometimes being able to ride with throttle power only?
- Do you have plenty of space for storage, or do you need to find a bike that can be folded when it's not in use?
- Do you want a regular bike, or a folding bike that you can take on transit?
- If you are thinking of a folding bike, how much weight can you comfortably lift on and off the bus or train?
- Do you want to be able to test ride the bike, or are you comfortable with mail order? Some bikes are only available via the Web. (Bear in mind that fit and comfort are very important. Personally I would never buy a bike without riding it first.)
- Would you prefer an electric bike that looks like a bike, or one that looks more like a scooter? Bear in mind that if you choose the latter, you are more likely to be pulled over by the police for not having registration on something that looks like a motorcycle. Also, this style bike can be dangerous because motorists may expect you to be able to go faster than you actually can. In general, it is probably better to have a vehicle that is faster than it looks, rather than one that is slower that it looks.

- Do you want to spend a decent chunk of money, or would you prefer a cheap bike? If your knee-jerk response is "cheap bike," bear in mind that a cheap bike will quickly fall apart, and the controller is likely to fail really soon.
- Think about what kinds of extras you want with your bike. Options include disc brakes, suspension, stand, lockable batteries, mudguards, rear carrier, front basket, lights, bell or horn. Some electric bikes come with a light and/or horn system powered by the primary battery. This can be a great option for safety, as it results in powerful lights and horn. Some of these options are non-negotiable – for example, riding a bike in the rain without fenders is a totally miserable experience. The last time I did it, I ended up with mud on my entire body, including my hair! A rear carrier is also pretty much a must-have: you don't want to be carrying luggage in a backpack like a school kid – it would not be comfortable or practical. You need a rear carrier to attach good quality panniers. Which reminds me – you will also need to buy accessories for your bike, such as panniers, and of course, a helmet.

With your answers to all of these questions fresh in your mind, you are ready to start evaluating the variety of bikes on offer.

One last caveat: once you do buy, check the bike really carefully before you take it home. Most electric bikes are made in China, and quality control varies widely. Often bikes are broken when shipped, so if the retailer has not checked the bike, you could be buying a broken bike. So try to make sure that you take home a bike that is not broken. Ride it at least around the block first. Also, try to make sure you are buying from a shop that offers good after-sales service.

Reviews of Selected Electric Bikes

A2B Electric Bike Review

This review reproduced with permission from NYCeWheels – New York's finest electric bike store.

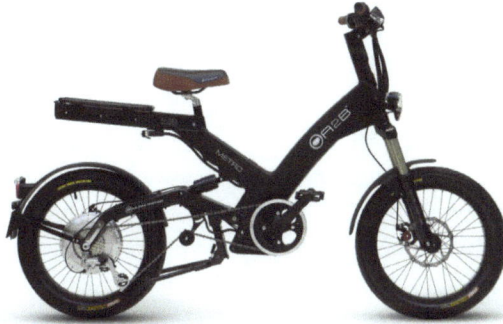

"Today definitely started the riding season. The forecast called for a 90 degrees high so I decided to take the A2B electric bike out for a good spin. We actually hit a record high of 92 degrees – the hottest since 1942.

I packed my Nikon SLR camera and headed towards the shop on York avenue to pick up the A2B. To my surprise, it was plugged in, fully charged (after a hectic Saturday, things usually are left as they come back from test drives).

With Austrian folk songs blasting from my MP3 player, I started going east on 85th street. The streets were not as bad as they were after recent winters in NYC, but I did hit a bad block on 3rd avenue. These potholes really showed off the front and rear suspension and wide tires of the A2B – it's smooth like Jaegermeister.

Arriving at Central Park, I parked the A2B electric bike at the baseball field just north of the great lawn. About 10 by-passers interrupted me, inquiring about the electric bike while shooting pictures, some of them pretty girls in bikinis, so it wasn't all that bad.

After finishing the 20-minute photo session, I kept going further east. I know you're not suppose to do this, but I took the A2B off-road to see how it handles in extreme riding. Well, I am impressed. I would not do a 12 foot drop off a cliff but dirt roads, paths through the woods and grass fields are right up its alley – what a pleasure.

After shooting another round of pictures on the west side of Central Park, I am entering Park Drive South and start heading home. I get flagged down a few more times. Although I am very handsome, I must admit I was mostly stopped because of the A to B electric bike.

I see my fuel-gauge still shows more than half a charge. I figure, why go home with a half-full battery? So I did another loop to finish off this perfect spring day in Central Park. Having tested pretty much every electric bike ever built, I must say the A2B is one of the most fun machines I have ever ridden. It's the most fun you could have going from A to B. "

BionX Electric Bike Kits Review

The BionX electric bike kit is reputed to be the best electric bicycle motor. It is certainly one of the most expensive. The company has been around for more than ten years, going from success to success, and claim to have a quarter of a million satisfied customers worldwide. I can only speak for one of these satisfied customers (me) – they are excellent systems that hold up to monsoon-like rain, snow, heat, and sub-zero conditions. Made in Quebec, Canada these kits come in a range of power options, and have a full two-year warranty. (I have had excellent experiences with this warranty.)

The best thing about these kits is that you can just buy one and retrofit a bike you already have. So if you already have an excellent bike and don't want to pay for a new bike with an electric assist, consider this option. They are powerful and noiseless, enabling you to infuriate younger cyclists by breezing past them on uphills!

The BionX system comprises a brushless hub engine, a

console on which you can choose four levels of positive or negative assistance (the latter for regenerating), a throttle control, and a lithium battery. The console allows you to select from 4 levels of positive energy and 4 levels of regenerative charging (for downhills).

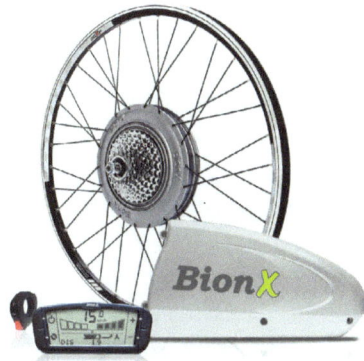

You can have a bike shop install a BionX kit for you (at a cost), or you can do it yourself. You could also buy a BionX system pre-installed on some bikes. A large number of bike companies have partnered with BionX to produce electric ranges. These include BiXS, DB Rent, Derby, Diamant, Focus, HP Velotechnik, Kalkhoff, Kilowatt, Klever, KTM, Matra, MS Design, Müsing, Mustang, OHM, Opus, Orbea, Oxford, Pro Aktiv, Riese & Müller, Raleigh, Rose, Smart, Steppenwolf, Stevens, Toba, Trek, Univega, Urbana, Viliger, and Wheeler. The reviews I have read of these partnership-based bikes have ranged from good to excellent.

On the negative side, these systems are not cheap, and neither are their batteries. It's the old story of you get what you pay for. In general, this applies to all electric bikes (and to bikes in general): the cheap ones are cheap for a reason; the good ones are not cheap, but they're good quality. However, bear in mind that there are some electric bikes out there that are expensive but are not good quality. At least with BionX, you get what you pay for.

BionX bike conversion kits are one of the few to use a proportional torque sensor. This basically means that it can magically figure out how hard you are pedaling, and match it. I have no idea how it does this, considering that half the time, I don't even know how hard I'm pedaling ... but still, I can vouch for the fact that it definitely does it, reliably, every time.

BionX PL-350 Review

The BionX PL-350 system is perfect kit for anyone who is challenged in their biking. The BionX PL-350 system offers a way to keep on cycling, and that's a beautiful thing.

Remember how we all wanted to be superheroes when we were kids? Well, when I first used a BionX electric bike system, it was like all those childhood dreams of being a superhero had finally come true. Even though it was just a bottom-of-the-range PL-250 BionX electric bike, my legs were suddenly bionic, and I could fly up hills with the greatest of ease. I went instantly from lagging behind, or not biking at all (I had been having some health problems) to metaphorically flying along, even overtaking younger people on uphills.

My Secret Superpower

The cool thing is that as the BionX electric bike system is so silent, people often don't even realize you have an assist. Especially as the engine is hidden in the back wheel, so that, as you can see in this photo, the fact that you have an assist is not blatantly obvious.

My Devinci Copenhagen with Bionx PL-350 kit

Sure, I had a secret, unfair advantage – but so do ALL superheroes. Comes with the territory – trust me, I know my superheroes.

Two years ago saw new challenges, when a different health issue reared its ugly head, **and** my commute changed to include a massive hill. My doctor approved the commute provided I had all the help I could get. So I upgraded to the PL-350 BionX electric bike kit, which has a much higher torque, and much more power.

BionX bills the BionX 350 electric bike as "the best in class for climbing, long rides and fast accelerations" – and that's absolutely true. Yet it is even more silent than the BionX 250 electric bike, so that I can still keep my superpower secret from many as I zoom up hills.

BionX Electric Bikes – a Truly Great System

Bottom line is that the BionX PL-350 electric bike kit is a GREAT system. You basically just retrofit your existing bike with a new back wheel (which has the motor built in), a large battery, and a console to control it all. (Well, in my case, I paid a bike shop to retrofit it.)

You still have the great feel of regular biking (although the bike is a lot heavier). And you can cycle without assist whenever you want, such as on flats (although in reality I almost never do that, because I love the extra speed I can get with the engine).

You can also choose from a huge variety of bikes that are already fitted with an integrated BionX engine – such as the Prodeco Phantom Folding Electric Bicycle.

Advantages of Having a BionX PL-350 Electric Bike Kit

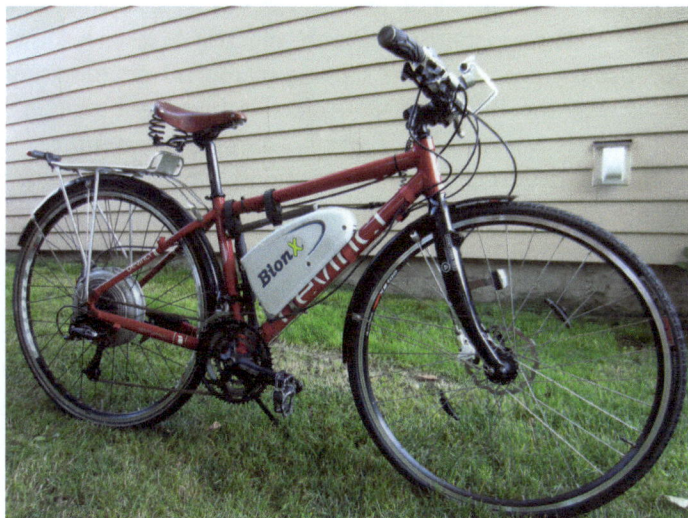

Make no mistake, I am still pedaling, and building up a sweat – I just go a WHOLE lot faster than I would without the BionX PL-350 electric bike. So the system is helping me build up my fitness, health and strength, and this is really apparent when I ride my regular bike on the weekend. I am now overtaking MUCH younger cyclists without an assist!

Also – and this is perhaps the greatest advantage – I bike much more often than I would if I did not have the BionX PL-350 electric bike kit. I really don't think I could face that huge hill twice a day, every day, without the BionX electric bike – it would just be too daunting. But with the BionX PL-350 electric bike, it's fun. Plus on the BionX PL-350 electric bike I can be at work in 35 minutes, as opposed to an hour or more on the bus.

Another advantage is that after the initial really large outlay, it's very, very cheap to run. The electricity it takes to charge is so minor I cannot even detect in on my electricity bill.

Bottom Line on the BionX PL-350 electric bike kit

I have ridden this bike non-stop through two rainy Vancouver winters, and even once got caught in snow. When that happened the BionX electric bike saved me, because my gears starting slipping so much I could hardly move, but the BionX PL-350 electric bike kept right on going like it was nothing (it was born in Montreal, after all).

I would unreservedly recommend the BionX PL-350 to anyone who is challenged in their biking by either very long distances, very steep terrain, or any kind of health issues. It's a way to keep on biking, and that's a beautiful thing.

BionX PL-250 Review

A BionX PL-250 kit can transform your bike into an electric bike in just one hour. Suddenly, you'll be able to bike faster and further than ever before!

I decided to get a BionX electric bike kit after experiencing some health problems that stopped me from doing strenuous activities for a while. Retrofitting my trusty Devinci commuter bike with a BionX PL-250 electric bike kit seemed like the perfect solution.

The Promised Benefits of the BionX PL-250 Electric Bike Kit

The cost was a bit intimidating – but the rewards promised to be great. I would be able to travel in an environmentally friendly way for pennies a day, while boosting my cardiac health, because the BionX electric bike kit merely assists – the cyclist still has to peddle. So I went ahead and ordered the Bionx electric bike kit from my friendly bike shop. I asked them to install it as well.

Anyone half-way handy can install the BionX kit personally; it's definitely not rocket science. Essentially it involves replacing the bike wheel (which houses the engine), putting the battery bracket on the down tube, mounting the control console on the handlebars, and connecting up the cabling (so that the brakes can function as cut-off devices, and to connect the battery input to the wheel). But I am only quarter-way handy, so I decided to pay for an hour of bike shop time.

Test Driving the BionX PL-250

Then came the happy day that I got to test drive my new electric bike. Before I set off, I had fully charged the rather heavy battery, just by plugging it into a wall socket. I slid the battery onto its mount, and locked it down. I have had problems with the BionX mounting on other bikes, but not on this particular bike.

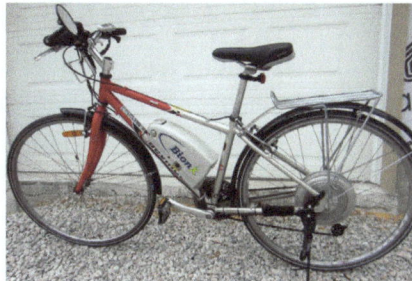

I set off from my (then) home in East Vancouver, en route to my (then) fiancée's condo in New Westminster, equipped with a large map, as I had never done this route before. My first ride with a BionX electric bike turned out to be a joyful experience. I have dreamed of being a superhero since I read my first

Superman comic at age five, and it had finally happened. With the BionX PL-250 electric bike I was suddenly Bionic Biker, fairly flying up hills with the greatest of ease. It was exhilarating! Suddenly I could really imagine giving up my family van and embracing an environmentally friendly transport form. Also, the BionX electric bike system is SILENT, so most people did not know I had an assist!

I felt like a GREEN WARRIOR!

How the BionX PL-250 Electric Bike Kit Works

The BionX electric bike kit utilizes a battery that charges a motorized back wheel.

It offers a choice of four levels of assistance, as well as a throttle on a handle-bar mounted console, for an extra boost when needed (useful when pulling off).

Pedalling is required, and the amount of assistance provided is proportionate to the amount of effort you put in – the harder you pedal, the more it will help you out. You can also switch to zero assistance on flats and downhills.

To prolong battery life, braking recharges the battery. Also, you can choose from four levels of resistance on downhills, which saves your brakes while at the same time charging the battery.

In short, the whole system is quite brilliant – a triumph of clever engineering that I would say justifies its steep price.

I pedalled along happily for a while, going much faster than usual on uphills, and saving the battery on all the flats. Although the BionX electric bike kit adds a hefty 30 pounds to a bike, it is still perfectly easy to pedal it on muscle power alone on flats. During the ride I was hit by a torrential downpour of rain, but the BionX kept on going like it was nothing at all. The BionX electric bike was a dream. It kept going the whole time, unperturbed by the pelting, soaking rain.

My love affair with electric bikes had begun, and it will last for the rest of my life.

The BionX electric bike unit was completely waterproof. In fact, I have ridden BionX electric bikes in pelting rain, day after day, and even in snow, without ever having a problem. One day my drive chain and gears froze and I could not pedal, but the BionX engine got me to work!

The BionX PL-250 electric bike did all I needed it to do. It got me cycling again, and it got me healthy and fit again (research shows that people with electric bikes often get fitter than people with regular bikes, because they bike more often). Eventually my commute changed to include very steep, very long hills, and I upgraded to a BionX PL-350 electric bike (although I still kept my PL-250 electric bike as a backup). Together, my two BionX electric bike kits have got me so fit that I now routinely bike 50 or 60 km a day on the weekend, without an assist.

My advice: if you need an assist and have a route that does not include monstrous hills, the BionX PL-250 electric bike should suffice to transform you from a car driver into a Green Warrior on a bike, leaving younger, fitter cyclists watching your disappearing tail lights and wondering what happened!

Bionx After-Sales Service

I love BionX products, and I was really happy to discover that their after sales service is almost as good as their products.

Rear Axle Blues

As I was riding my brown BionX Pl-350 electric bike one day, the rear axle snapped clean in half. This was the axle that is supplied by BionX, as part of the motorized back wheel.

This was not a fun incident.

I was pretty well flummoxed. I had been commuting

on BionX bikes for six years by then, and this was the first time I had a major problem. I knew I had a major problem because my electric bike suddenly became wobbly, and the BionX pretty much stopped working. It was time to get off my bike and call for help.

Which I did. My wife Maggie (Mrs. Average Joe Cyclist) quickly rescued me, and I was soon in the bike shop that sold me my BionX – the Bike Doctor. They quickly diagnosed a snapped-in-half rear axle. Not the kind of thing you fix with a band aid.

Long story short: the Bike Doctor organized for BionX to replace the back wheel – free of charge, even though the BionX kit was already two years old, and I could not find my receipt. Given that the rear wheel houses the entire engine, I now had a completely new engine. I was really impressed by this excellent service, from both the Bike Doctor and BionX.

Problems with my BionX Battery Mount

It was apparently my season for BionX problems, because a short time later, my down-tube mounted battery became so wobbly that it was clearly unsafe to ride. Back to Bike Doctor I went.

After removing the battery mount, it was clear I had a serious problem. There were gaping, ragged holes in the frame, apparently caused by wobbling battery mount screws. It was so bad that the frame was compromised.

I was pretty distraught. My bike is a Devinci Copenhagen, and it was not cheap. I have it fully outfitted for commuting to work, so all in all it is a pretty sweet bike. That I happen to love. Even though it is brown (I chose the bike on its merits, but I was not bowled over by its paint job).

Pol at the Bike Doctor stepped up to bat for me. He called Devinci and BionX, and between the two of them he managed to broker a very acceptable deal for me.

Devinci didn't want to replace the frame outright, because they said it was never meant to hold a BionX battery. However, they were prepared to offer me a replacement frame at a cut-rate price.

BionX wasn't really interested in helping me, because it was the Devinci frame that died, not their product. However, BionX's new Canadian distributor, Cycles Lambert, apparently took pity on me, and agreed to pay for the cut-rate frame offered by Devinci. And I was also able to buy a matching fork for a cut-rate price. Finally, the Bike Doctor rebuilt the bike and re-fitted the battery (and all my accessories) for a really good price.

All in all, I now have an almost entirely new bike for relatively very little financial outlay.

But here's the sweetest part – the new frame is RED! I've always wanted a red bike, and now I finally have one. Maggie picked the bike up from the shop for me, and when she came home bearing a red bike, it was like Christmas in October!

All in all, pretty good after-sales from both Devinci and BionX, plus skillful, customer-focused negotiation from Pol at the Bike Doctor, means that I was a happy electric bike commuter again!

In retrospect, I realize that when I bought my BionX, the seller never showed me how to gently remove the battery, so I had been a bit rough with it. This problem should not happen to you if you are gentle.

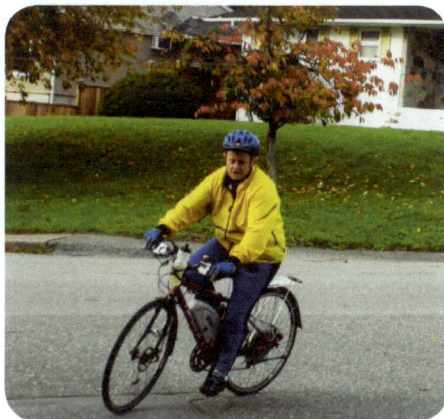

Brompton Electric Folding Bike Review

This review reproduced with permission from NYCeWheels – New York's finest electric bike store.

This is a nice guest review by our happy customer, Steve H. I've inserted a few comments when appropriate to address some of his thoughts and questions. – Peter, NYCeWheels MD.

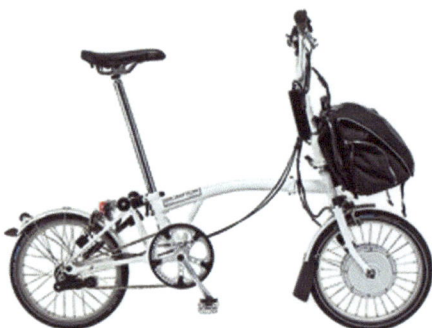

Just returned from our boat trip to Canada. Sarah and I rode about 60 miles (she has a trip computer). That is more than I have cycled in YEARS. My wife was DELIGHTED I had the electric Brompton because it let her bike at her usual all out she-woman pace and I could easily stay with her or catch up with a burst of "warp mode." What I really found was that the bike allowed me to maintain flat road conditions at all times, letting me pedal and get exercise without showing my age and having a coronary. As the hills came on I eased on some volts to reduce my pedaling effort. The bike was much admired at various stops.

I never saw the charge light go down by even one "red" after two or three hours. Don't know if the battery is just so great or if the lights are not all that accurate. Never lost any juice in half day rides. Charged it each time which took several hours.

Peter: Steve's 15 AH battery is very large capacity and should last him 30 to 40 miles of riding with pedaling.

Love that the HEAVY front bag is mounted on the stem and not on the handle bars which would be really dangerous. The weight always stays centered. A really good feature.

The bag holds a ton of stuff and is very well designed. I would like a rear bag or rack but don't know if they make it or if it would interfere with folding. Peter: you can get a rack and a bag for it too, the bike folds just fine with these attached.

The old fart seat I bought was a good decisions. No "SA" (sore ass) even after two straight hours biking.

I was thinking it would be nice for there to be an easy to mount/remove main tube clip (between the legs) to hold spare battery. I would buy a 10 AH spare just to have it. I always expect the worst. :)

The bike is just great. At first I had a problem of getting the front wheel hook up over the tube to release it but now I've got the trick down. Slow learner.

Currie IZIP Zuma Review

This review reproduced with permission from NYCeWheels – New York's finest electric bike store – and with permission from Turbo Bob, one of the greatest online electric bike reviewers. I highly recommend his blog, which you can find at https://turbobobbicycleblog.wordpress.com/

When it comes to beach cruising E-bikes the IZIP E3 Zuma is king. Yet part of the fun of any beach cruiser is the chance to find the snazzy color combo that matches your style. With the new 2013 line-up of IZIP E3 Zumas you can find the shade that suits your fancy and E-bike your way to comfort and happiness.

Tucked down inside the rear wheel is the quiet and powerful 500 watt motor. Controlled automatically with

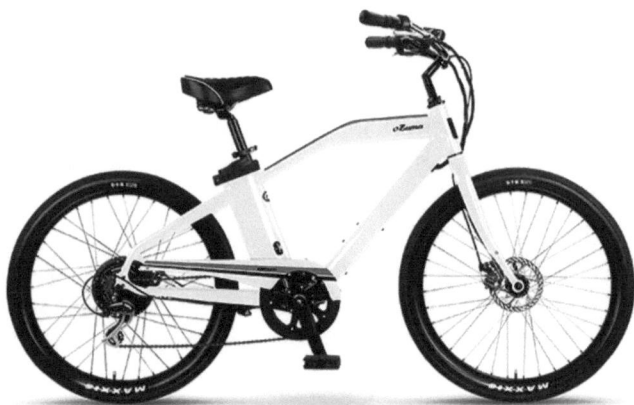

the PAS system or manually by a twist throttle, it will propel you into strong winds and up those nasty hills with no noise or strain. Of course these are the main reasons you are considering this new E-bike. If you want you can motor along without pedaling, yet your feet will turn the pedals anyway, it's only natural.

The strong beefy aluminum cantilever frame comes in two styles, diamond and low. Nowhere in this bike will you find anything that says wimpy. Don't think of the two frames as gender specific, think more about rider size. I have long called low-framed bikes comfort step-through bikes. Plus in the different frames you will find varying colors. So when picking the E3 Zuma you want, think color charts and your stature. Try both bikes to see which one fits you the best.

The IZIP E3 Zuma I've been riding is the low-framed model. I chose that one so my wife could ride it easily, yet my 6'2" body fits on it fairly well. I also like to let any and all interested parties try out the bikes I test, so I thought it was a good choice in that respect too. I've also ridden the larger one and found it is more my size, but never once did the low-frame bike cramp my style. Pick your color and go from there.

Even though the Zuma is a cruiser, there is plenty of speedster lurking under the hood. You can tool around with a smile or bear down on the pedals and motor with gusto. It has the ability to take your biking mood and make it fly. When you are flying on this E-bike you might be happy to know that a big set of disc brakes are there to back you up. Anytime the need arises, a quick pull on the handbrakes will satisfy your stopping desires. Yes they look cool too.

With the large capacity (11.4 Ah) 36 volt battery you should enjoy the longest of powered range. I took many rides in the 30 to 40 miles distance and never ran short of power. Yet with the way this bike is designed, non-powered riding is quite fun. My wife, who likes the exercise function of bikes, did many of her rides with the electric-assist turned off. It was there for the hills and the such, but she enjoyed the smooth pedaling it offered on many of the rides we took.

This is one thing I test on all the E-bikes I ride. Seeing that an E-bike should be all bike (with that one added accessory – the boost), I always make sure they act and ride like an everyday bicycle. There are some you would be hard pressed to pedal without power, you will find that the IZIP E3 Zuma is not one of them. It has a full selection of gears, including the extra low first gear, that make riding fun and easy. Shifting is a breeze too.

So pick your colors, mount your steed and enjoy the world from the saddle of this awesome E-bike, Turbo Bob.

Dahon Folding Electric Bike Review – Dahon Matrix with Bionx PL-350

This review reproduced with permission from NYCeWheels – New York's finest electric bike store.

When Bert first proposed I take an electric bike home to test drive, my immediate thought was: "I'm subletting in the smallest apartment in Brooklyn. I don't even think I can fit an electric bike through the door." With a basement apartment, this required carrying the bike up and down a pretty narrow flight of stairs. This is something I didn't want to risk on a $1800 bike.

Enter the Dahon Matrix. Full size mountain bike. Compact folding bike. Bionx PL-350 system installed. This seemed like the best option. It only folded in half, but this was enough to get it through the narrow stairs with little effort.

So I took off from NYCeWheels on the Matrix and was immediately impressed with the suspension. Since

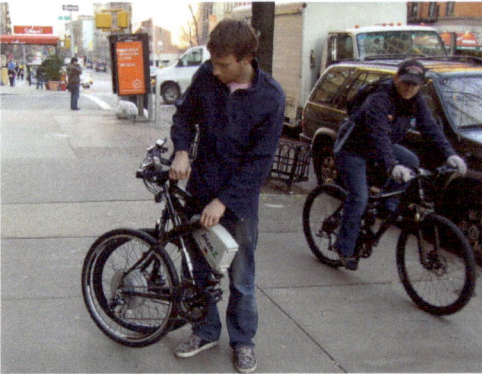

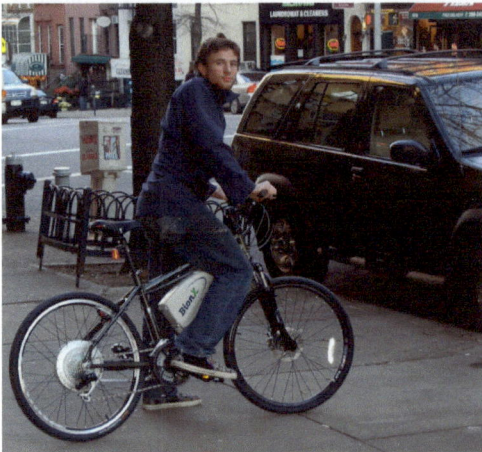

the Matrix is a mountain bike, it can handle the potholes and imperfections of my terribly bumpy Second Avenue commute. The bike handled well, it felt just like a mountain bike. Compared to any other folding bike, this frame felt a lot sturdier. With two locking Allen key bolts, this also locks together better than any other folding bike.

The Bionx electric motor kit, at a hefty 20 lbs, added some noticeable weight to the bike. Although this could be seen as a setback, I soon found out why. The power in the PL-350 with a 36 Volt battery was enormous! I set the Pedal Assist to 2, meaning 50% additional power. I coasted through traffic with ease. When I needed a boost to get around a car or a quick jump when stopped at a red light, the throttle option (300% power boost) was fantastic. The stop-and-go process can really be exhausting when traffic lights turn green and bikers have to start pedaling from a stop. With the throttle, I could now get up to speed with traffic about ten times faster. This was one of the best things about the BionX system.

The throttle was impressive, and it will obviously drain the battery much quicker than a simple pedal-assist. However, I used the throttle quite liberally in my 9-mile commute to Brooklyn and found that I still had about half the battery life remaining. This may be due to the regeneration option on the BionX. Instead of using pedal-assist, the BionX allows for a resistance mode, which actually charges the battery while you ride. This is similar to riding an exercise bike with added resistance. As you pedal downhill, the resistance charges the battery. Additionally, the rear brake can be used at any time to trigger this same option. Switching between assist and regeneration modes, I found it easy to extend the battery life for a long time.

In the end, the Bionx system made my commute super easy. I could make it from the Upper East Side to Brooklyn and barely break a sweat. It was also very simple to learn, with a few easy-to-use buttons on the controller. For a folding electric bike, the Matrix really felt like a durable and helpful investment.

EcoBike Vatavio Review

This review reproduced with permission from NYCeWheels – New York's finest electric bike store.

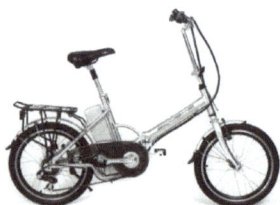

The EcoBike Vatavio can be deceptively meek looking but don't be fooled. This step-through electric folding bike has a lot of power despite its compact appearance.

I got to ride an EcoBike Vatavio all over the Upper East Side a few days ago and man was it fun. The small wheels mean quick and responsive handling that's perfect for getting around in the city. You can duck right around pot holes and cracks, easily slip between parked cars, and when it's time to go to work you just fold it up and lock it up. Because it folds you can put a chain all the way through the whole frame and wheels so it's much harder for thieves to take anything.

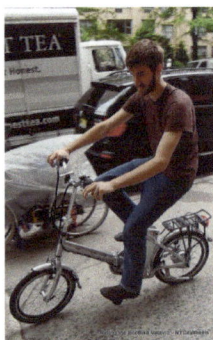

It's not just my experience with this EcoBike that made me raise my eyebrows, other people have been having great success with this compact electric bike too. There is one woman who bought her EcoBike Vatavio midway through the summer of 2010 who has been riding it 27 miles a day on a single charge! 27! That's quite a boastful range for such a little electric bike. It's all made possible by the combination of a pedelec and throttle based drive system.

The EcoBike Vatavio has 3 modes. You can ride it like a regular bike with no motor resistance, this is regular bike mode. You can ride it with a % 50 motor assistance, this is pedelec mode. Lastly, you can use the throttle on the right side for a boost up hills and on start ups. The combination of these three modes really allows you to choose how much you want to work or how much you want the motor to work for you. Tired of riding? Scoot home on the throttle. Want to get some light exercise on the way to work without getting soaked in sweat? Use the pedelec mode and save the throttle as an additional boost when you need it. Want to just go out and ride a normal bike? Turn the electric system off, that way you can pedal as usual.

With this compact electric folding bike you get a little bit of everything. It's a great bike for daily use or weekend leisure rides. Check out the EcoBike Vatavio electric bike. It's one powerful electric bike in one small package.

eFlow Nitro Electric Bike Review

This review reproduced with permission from NYCeWheels – New York's finest electric bike store.

This is Jeremy here with a review of the eFlow Nitro, a powerful electric bicycle from Currie Technologies. I just had the privilege of test riding one of these amazing bikes and have a lot to share about my experience with it. To start off, the eFlow bike is a large bicycle. I am a 5'11" rider and had to do a little bit of a jump to get on and situated. Once on I had absolutely no idea of the thrilling trip I was about to embark on. One of the first things that becomes evident is that the eFlow Nitro helps you along the way. While pedaling you will feel the back wheel automatically giving you that extra boost. This feature is especially beneficial in getting you around faster and with extreme ease.

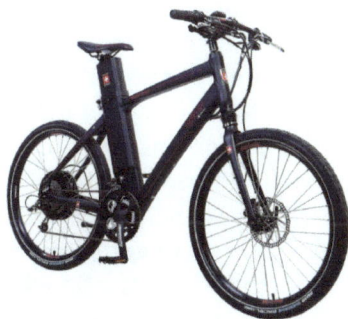

Speed and Stopping Power

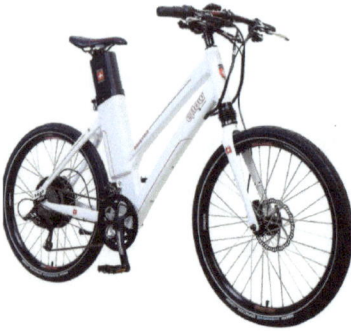

While you have the traditional option of using the pedals with that extra kick, you also get the handlebar throttle which works like a motorcycle when twisted, so the electric bike zooms you forward without any need for pedaling. I decided to test both features out and see how they differ by cycling uphill through Central Park all the way to its northernmost edge at 110th street. With my hands freezing from the windchill, I felt like I was flying as I sped on up the hills and barreled around the park's wide turns.

eFlow Electric bike computer

And speaking of speed, the hand brakes on the eFlow Nitro are spot on. No matter how fast you are flying through the wind or downhill, the moment you pull on the breaks the eFlow

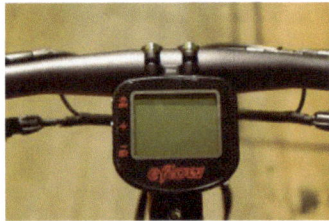

Nitro comes to a complete stop without any skidding. This proved to be a great help when riding through thick traffic on narrow streets. With vehicles constantly stopping and starting without warning, it felt excellent to be able to do the same and stop abruptly as needed. This combination of speed and stopping power makes the eFlow one of the best electric bikes for commuting.

Comfortable, Beautiful, Powerful

The eFlow is equipped with a small digital computer that tracks your distance traveled as well as your miles per hour during your entire ride. It was nice to be able to quickly look down while riding and see exactly how fast I was going and how much distance I had covered in such a short amount of time. A few other great things about the eFlow electric bike include its highly comfortable geometry, handsome black matte aesthetic, and buttery eFlow adjustable suspension – smooth ride even when trekking down bumpy debris covered paths. The adjustable suspension fork and cushy hand grips are great at absorbing some of the shock you may encounter on larger dips and bumps, so riding the eFlow Nitro felt like flying through the clouds.

The eFlow Nitro's battery rests right below the seat which keeps it balanced and stable, and is also easily removable for charging. While riding you will always feel the power right beneath you and all throughout the build of this amazing and beautifully designed machine. I would highly recommend this bicycle to anyone that is looking to get around faster, that has a need to tackle uneven terrain and steep hills, and even to anyone just looking for a fun, exhilarating and intense bicycle to explore with.

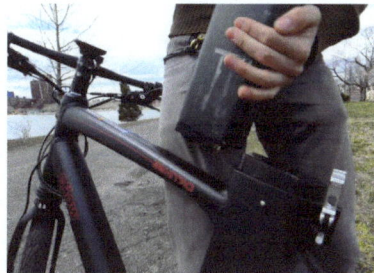

The Currie Technologies eFlow Nitro electric bike is the complete package: functionality, style, and strength united to make a truly fun bicycle.

eFlow E3 Nitro Review
by Turbo Bob

This review reproduced with permission from NYCeWheels – New York's finest electric bike store – and with permission from Turbo Bob, one of the greatest online electric bike reviewers. I highly recommend his blog, which you can find at https://turbobobbicycleblog.wordpress.com/

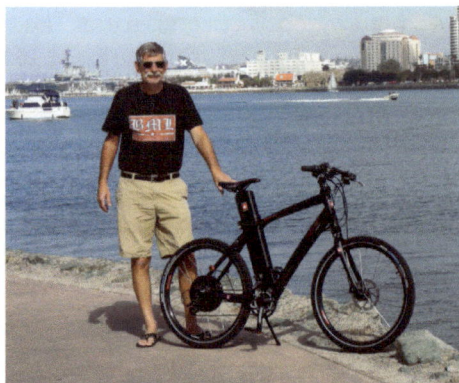

I just got the word that NYCeWheels has taken delivery of the brand new eFlow E3 Nitro electric-assist bike. This great piece of engineering was just released this month and is really spec'd nicely. I was at the introduction that took place at the 2013 Interbike Electric Bike Media Event on the 13th. What was even cooler is that I got to take one of the demo bikes home to ride for a month or two. So stay tuned for all the skinny on this and other electric bikes.

Features of the eFlow Nitro electric bike

This E3 Nitro has all the new stuff. With load-sensed pedelec, it knows what you want and how to deliver. With a very quick computer running the motor, you are assured of a fun and exhilarating ride. The bike looks good, is kind of stealthy, and has a very sport tuned chassis. The gearing, wheels and tires and the whole layout has been worked to perfection for you and me.

From the front, you find a large disc brake that works with hydraulics, not a cable. It is very capable of its chores as you pound the roadways. Smooth, strong and powerful are just a few words to describe the braking system on the eFlow. They mounted-up a set of tires I am quite pleased with. They have a large cross-section that is easy rolling and soaks up the bumps well too. The alloy rims are black and appear to be as beefy as need be.

A uni-shock front suspension locates the front end. It has a pre-load adjustment that took a few tries on the setting to match-up to my riding style and now feels just right. As I work the ruts and bumps, I feel very confident when the speeds ramp-up. The frame geometry has a sport feel with good feed-back that I am enjoying very much. With a semi-aggressive riding position, you are at the right angle for all types of riding. The short, fairly straight bars on the eFlow electric bike have room for all my lights and goodies.

E3 Nitro bike design and battery

Part of the difference of this eFlow is the battery being in the seat post. It blends in well with the frame and puts the weight (which isn't that much) right in line with that of the rider. It is easy to remove the battery if you like, and it can be charged on or off the bike depending on your needs. It slides up and down for the saddle height adjustment and has a spot by the quick release clamp for a small padlock if you think it is necessary to secure the seat and the battery to the bike. Mounted on top is a racy saddle that, although it felt good, I swapped out for one a little wider.

This E3 Nitro electric bike comes with a removable display unit. It can be set and reviewed when off the bike due to an internal coin battery. The bike's power system is disabled when the computer is removed as a security tool. The display reads out the speed, other bike computer functions and your power assist sensitivity levels. It also has small indicators that read out the amps used and regenerated during your ride.

A multi-speed drive train is found under your feet as you pedal. With two gears in front and ten in the rear, that adds up to twenty available at your disposal. Everything is run with SRAM Apex derailleurs and thumb shifters. You can blast through the gears like a pro and ride this bike just fine without the power-assist if you want. But when you want some power, it is at the ready to help you up the hills, into a head wind and if you are just plain tuckered out after a long blast of electric assist bike fun.

Riding the eFlow Nitro bicycle

The motor on the eFlow Nitro is whisper-quiet and more powerful than you really need. The power comes on seamlessly, just like load-sensor pedelec should. You can override the intelligent pedelec at any time with a twist of the half-hand throttle. The power-system is well thought out and works with you, not against you. What more could you want than that? The frame comes with all the places and fittings you need to add bags or racks for some major touring. I added all kinds of goodies from a local bike accessory supplier to make mine more fun, safer and to add utility. You can check the video on my YouTube channel or my bike blog (https://turbobobbicycleblog.wordpress.com/) to learn all about those. I do recommend adding lights and the such to your new eFlow E3 Nitro before you ride it home.

So contact NYCeWheels to see what all the fuss is about. The eFlow E3 Nitro is new, rides great and might be the one you've been waiting for. Look for more from me as I continue to put this super machine through its paces.

eFlow with the road, Turbo Bob.

Emotion Neo City
Electric Bike Review

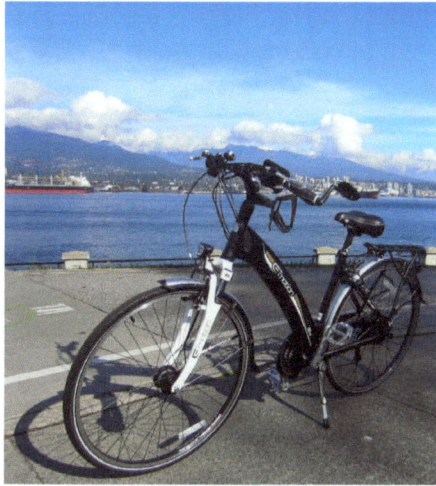

The Easy Motion Neo City from BH is an ideal bike for bike commuters, especially if your commute is challenging – for example if you are dealing with hills, long distances, or rough urban roads and bike trails full of potholes. And because it's so comfy, it's perfect if you just want to get on your bike and ride, without putting on Lycra.

The bike has Suntour front shocks with 62 mm of travel; big wheels (29") and smooth-rolling Kenda puncture-resistant tires; a comfort saddle with springs; and offers a relaxed upright riding position. The stem has a quick release device that allows you to adjust the handle bars to exactly the most comfortable position for you (no tools or techie expertise required!)

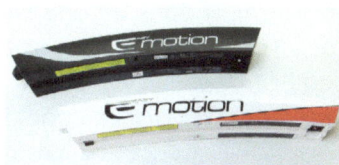

The lines are sleek, and the styling is integrated and efficient. The battery (a Lithium-ion Samsung with 36 volts and 9 amp hours) is cunningly integrated into the down tube, making for a slightly more "stealth" electric bike look, and a balanced weight distribution (necessary on a bike that weighs in at 52 pounds for the medium size, 55 pounds for the large). This is the kind of stylish integration that people have come to expect from the manufacturers of the Emotion bikes – a company called BH, located in Spain. They have been making bikes for more than a hundred years, and it shows.

The 350 watt geared engine is controlled by a backlit, removable, CD computer console, conveniently mounted right next to your left thumb. This makes it very easy to change levels of assistance. There are four levels of assist. These are the power modes (that is, how much extra power you get for each push at the pedals):

Ride Mode: 70% extra power in each turn of the pedal (Economy)

Trip Mode: 140% extra power in each turn of the pedal (Standard)

Sport Mode: 200% extra power in each turn of the pedal (Sport)

Fast Mode: Triple the power in each turn of the pedal (Boost)

One of the best things about this bike is that it also has a zero level of assist. First, this means you can switch into serious exercise mode without having to power down the motor. Second, you have the option of using the throttle assist when you are in zero level assist.

When I test rode this bike, I vividly remember the instant that I realized it had both throttle and pedal assist. That was the moment the giant "SOLD!" sign flashed in my brain. I love having both options on one bike. Previously I have ridden throttle-only and pedal-assist only, but never a bike that offered both. The beauty of this is that you can choose what works best for various conditions.

The pedal assist is the best for challenging hills, because it integrates the efficiency of a 24-speed drive-train with the power of a very torque-sensitive rear hub pedal assist motor (a 350 watt geared engine). And I do mean very sensitive. The minute you realize you're on a tough hill and put your feet to the metal, the engine gets on board with you and pounds out the power. Awesome!

The throttle assist is great for pulling off, and for sudden bursts of speed (like when a car is too close, or a traffic light is about to turn yellow). This is one of the great things about electric bikes – I believe they are safer than regular bikes, because you can put in a burst of amazing speed when you need to. I find I have the confidence to be in zero assist most of the time on this relatively heavy bike, because I know I can engage that throttle and be out of harm's way in a heartbeat. The throttle assist is also great for fine maneuvering at slow speed around obstacles and pedestrians.

The gears are controlled by rapid-fire shifters within easy reach, making it really easy to change the gears. And 24 gears makes it easy to use the bike with no assist at all. On the other hand, another option is that you can just cruise along without pedaling at all! You can easily do 32 km per hour on a flat road without pedaling at all, just using the throttle. When testing this mode, I was also surprised to find that you can keep going without pedaling over fairly substantial uphills (although of course you slow down). It is nice to have this option when you are tired or injured – or just want to sit back and feel the wind on your helmet!

Range: there are so many variables in electric bikes that this is a near-impossible question. Variables include terrain, weather, your weight, and how hard you pedal. The claimed range from the manufacturers is 50 miles (80 km), but I assume this is for someone who weighs 100 pounds, and is going downhill while pedaling hard! Seriously though, it does have an excellent range, just not as much as 50 miles – not for average cyclists, anyway. Like many electric bikes, the engine is capped at 32 km/20 miles per hour.

The battery takes between three and four hours to charge, depending on how much I have depleted it. Of course it is a smart battery, so you don't have to fully deplete it before charging.

Plus points: The frame is step-through, making it easy to get on – even when I have one of the injuries I seem to get more and more frequently, the older I get. The LCD computer console is removable for safe parking. I love the fact that this bike has both pedal assist AND throttle drive. It gives me all the options I need for my very challenging commute (which includes tight turns, steep hills, hill pull-offs, and traffic dodging).

The full accessories set is great: serious wrap-around fenders with mud flaps; chain guard; ergonomic grips; solid, rugged rear carrying rack; dynamo powered LED lights that stay on long after you stop pedaling; and adequate kickstand. All I had to buy were a bell and a rear-view mirror. The wires and cables are integrated into the frame so that they are safe. It is impossible to get caught without lights. The built-in lights (powered by a dynamo in the front hub) are quite powerful and very visible. The rear light is always on. The front light has an on/off switch. I leave it permanently on. I am not sure why anyone would want to switch off a free light on a bike. Even during the day, vehicles with lights are much more visible. That's why compulsory daytime lights for cars were introduced, after all. However, I don't think these lights are adequate for riding in pitch darkness.

Cons: It comes with mechanical V-brakes. Disk brakes would be better – apparently these will come standard with the 2015 Easy Motion Neo City. There is nowhere to put your water bottle. I bought a bottle cage that attaches to the stem with a strap.

The Emotion Neo City comes ready-to-ride, in a sleekly integrated commuter cyclist package. It's not like someone bought a bike and then decided to slap on an engine and some commuter accessories. It's brilliantly conceptualized right from the start as an electric commuter bike. To my mind, it's one of the best possible electric bikes for bike commuters, and the price point is excellent value for money. No wonder it's the best seller in the entire excellent Neo line.

Emotion Street 650
by Mrs. Average
Joe Cyclist (Maggie)

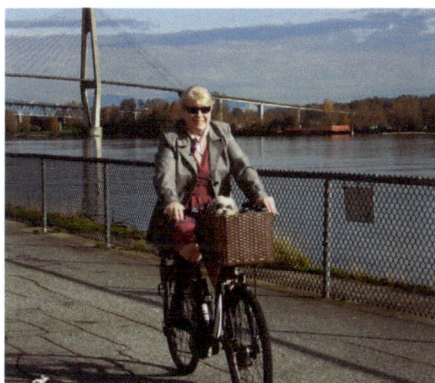

The Emotion Street 650 from BH is an ideal bike for women. I use it for commuting as well as weekend leisure rides and running errands. In July 2013 I changed jobs and my commute changed. Before, I rode my Giant Avail 3 on a relatively off road and level terrain. Now I had to travel a rough industrial and hilly ride. After a few trips on my Avail it became evident that one or both of us was not going to survive this commute. Out of love for my Avail, I retired it to weekend jaunts and charity rides such as the MS Bike Ride.

I had spent countless hours in Evolution Bikes in North Vancouver while Joe test drove a number of bikes, and talked endlessly with the owner Mark about the benefits of BH bikes versus Bionics kits and Panasonic versus Bosch engines…blah, blah, blah. However, on one trip I noticed the Emotion Street 650 and was curious enough to take a test drive of my own.

It took me about two minutes to fall in love with the Street 650. I had a vision of myself wearing a summer dress, large sunglasses, and a scarf…think Audrey Hepburn in Roman Holiday. I imagined myself meeting friends for a glass of wine, perhaps with one of our dogs in a front wicker basket.

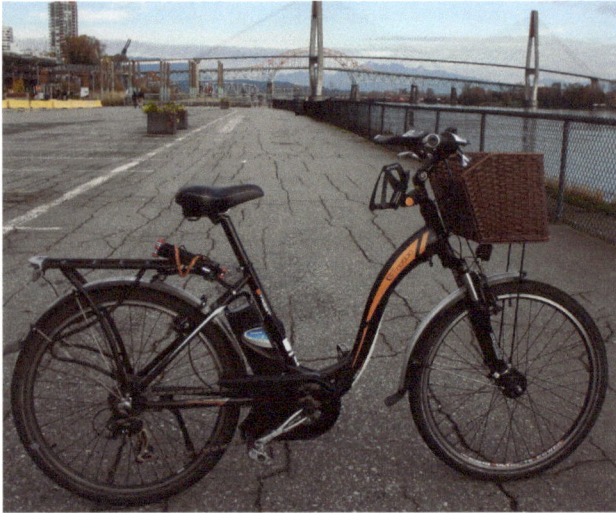

What can I say... she is gorgeous. Stylishly curved step-through frame, black with orange accents, integrated dynamo front and back lights, big comfy wide tires and super comfy saddle, front shocks, and custom rear bike rack. The motor lives in the drive train and the battery tucks nicely behind the down tube, next to the back tire. The battery is represented as having a range of approximately 40 km when new. This is dependent on so many factors that it is hard to verify. I can only confirm that I have never run out of power on any commute. Now that the battery is a year old, the range seems a little reduced but I still have not run out of power. I would put the range at around 25 km (16 miles). Best of all, the battery charges in a couple of hours, seated in a soundless floor charger unit.

The bike is much heavier than my racer, but it is surprisingly nimble. Despite weighing in at 50 lbs, the bike is easy to maneuver without battery power. I only bought my Easy Motion Street 650 because of the tough commute I was facing. I still wanted to improve my fitness. The Street 650 is pedal-assist technology which means that the motor only engages when you are pedaling. With 7 gears and 3 levels of assist, you have 21 optional settings to tackle any terrain the Lower Mainland can throw at you.

I am happy to report that I can still arrive at work sweaty and smelly…just the way I like it. (Note that I do shower before inflicting myself on my colleagues.)

The frame is step-through, making it easy to get on – even in a dress. I love the fact that this bike is pedal assist. Down with throttle drive! (Joe is spitting as I write this.) The bike is fully accessorized. I only bought a bottle cage and more ergonomic grips. The built-in lights (powered by a dynamo in the front hub)

The bikes comes with V-brakes which means they wear out a lot if you bike a lot. Which I do. I understand that some of the new models will come out with disk brakes – that will be better. There is no place to mount a water bottle except on the stem. Maybe it is the sort of bike you shouldn't need a water bottle for. But I ride it hard and need water. I have a cage mounted on the stem, but it is awkward. It does swivel so you can keep it out of the way of the step-through frame but I have had a couple of nasty scratches when pedaling if it moves into the path of my legs.

I paid just over $3,000 for this bike at Evolution Bikes in North Vancouver. Being an accountant, I have to mention the rationale of why I spent $3,000 on a bike. Factoring in that a transit ticket would cost me $170 per month (!!), the bike can be paid off in 18 months – and after riding it for about a year, my bike is still almost as good as new! I contrast my commute, rain or shine, by myself, in the outdoors, versus a crowded, smelly transit trip dependent on the transit system's schedule. My trip only takes 40 minutes on a bike, and would take over an hour on transit. So I'm saving time and money – while burning calories and getting fit! (And on transit I would risk getting sick too – transit riders are six times more likely to catch acute respiratory infections.)

Unlike Joe, I didn't do a lot of research before I bought. Quite frankly there was nothing remotely as stylish on the market. The Emotion Street 650 comes ready to ride with very few add-ons required. This is a great alternative to a crowded commuter train any time of the year!

Elite Electric Bikes

These bikes utilize the maximum size motor (500 watt) and battery (48 volt) currently legal in Canada. They use a Lithium Manganese (LiMg204) battery, which is the same battery technology used in the Nissan Leaf hybrid car. The manufacturers claim this setup can propel the bike up to 32 km/h carrying a 150 kg load for up to 60 km on a single charge. Doing some innovative marketing in *CGA Magazine*, they were offering a $150 discount to CGA members, and proclaiming that the bike will give a great roi (return on investment), due to savings in gas, car depreciation, and parking fees, so as to pay off the bike in less than a year.

However, these bikes are sold via online sales only, and when I emailed them to ask to borrow one to do a review, they ignored me, so I was less than impressed. Still, check it out for yourself: http://eliteelectricbikes.com/

eZee ForZa Review

This review reproduced with permission from NYCeWheels – New York's finest electric bike store. This review was written by Andrew K. in California.

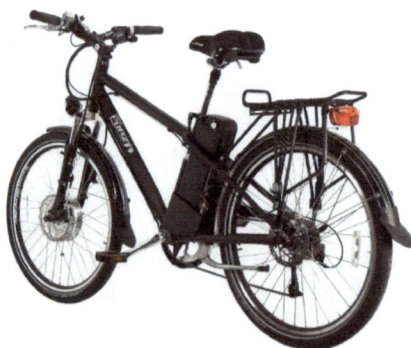

I recently bought an eZee ForZa electric bike because I intended to commute to work and get some exercise. I work at a laboratory in Pasadena. It is about a 9 mile ride for me by bicycle from San Marino where I live. It is

100% uphill to get there. Near the end of my trip I have to climb out of the Rose Bowl (for those of you familiar with the locality) up a street with a truly fierce grade. The Forza performed valiantly. The battery, of course, has to be recharged at work because the uphill ride is so power consuming.

On this bike, there is a control that allows you to choose the degree of pedal assist. It is not exactly a throttle, nothing happens until you pedal. By adjusting the pedal assist, you not only set the degree of exercise you get, but also indirectly determine the range. Less assist, more range. I find I can set it to get some decent exercise without sweating like a pig. As a result, I don't have to clean up when I get to work. This saves the inconvenience and a lot of time. When I used my conventional bike, I got more exercise, but I went only now and then. I use my Forza electric bike most days.

The eZee Forza is fast, at maximum assist you can do 20 mph, or about 14 mph up a steep hill. On long rides you may pass up maximum assist to extend the range. One thing to keep in mind is that near the end of charge you cannot attempt a long steep hill at full power because you will drive the battery indicator into the red zone. Some power management is required if you want to use the electric bicycle near its maximum range.

The eZee ForZa electric bike is a pleasing flat black in color and has puncture resistant 26" x 1.95 tires. The wide tires are great for a commute bike and the front fork shock absorbers and seat shock further improve the ride. It comes equipped with a speedometer/odometer, battery status indicator, a front and rear light. The rear light is quite bright, the front white LED light is only good for being spotted on a dark street. The tires have reflective material along the rim.

The brakes are excellent. The rear wheel has disk brakes and the front wheel has hydraulic brakes. The bicycle also has an 8 gear change which allows you to match your legs to the motor. It has a nice ratcheting lever actuation right on the handlebar.

The bicycle has two minor faults. The seat is designed to flip up to make battery removal easier. The mechanism used prevents the seat from tilting forward, a position I find more comfortable. This can be remedied by replacing the seat post with a conventional shock absorbing one for very little cost. Secondly, the electric motor engages when you pedal with a bit of delay. The delay is very short in low gear, but in high gear it can be significant. High gear is when the delay is least tolerable. I usually downshift when I get to a light.

Andrew K., San Marino, CA

Haibike Electric Mountain Bikes

This review reproduced with permission from NYCeWheels – New York's finest electric bike store.

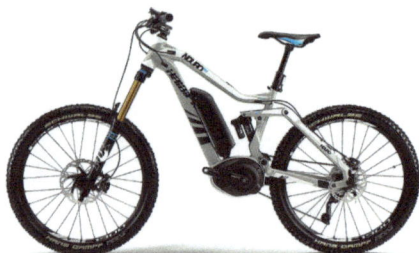

Whether you're a seasoned mountain bike rider looking for a little boost or a first time mountain biker finding yourself intimidated by steep hills and long wilderness trails, these Haibikes will allow you to conquer anything in your path. No matter where in the world you are, you will be able to finally enjoy some peace and quiet far from civilization. The Bosch center drive electric motor systems – integrated right into the frame of these high end mountain bikes – pack enough power to carry you wherever you desire.

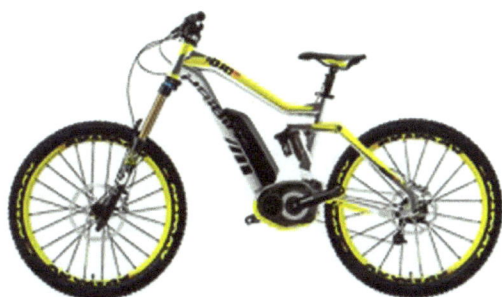

Haibike is already the number one non-electric mountain bike company in Germany and now that they've teamed up with Currie Technologies an entirely new monster has been born. These bikes combine quality Made In Germany manufacturing with Currie Tech's US Market support and experience. Each and every Haibike you order from NYCeWheels ships tuned-up and ready to ride so pick your bike, pick your trail, and get ready for a weekend you'll never forget!

What puts a Haibike ahead of the competition?

The Bosch Center drive Motor on these bikes delivers a silent and yet extremely powerful motor assist to augment your pedaling. By working through the gears of the bike's drivetrain the motor is able to achieve a better distribution of torque throughout all speeds. Because of this heightened efficiency the bicycles are also quite light weight – ranging between just 45 and 50 lbs. Plus, with the motor and battery literally centered in the frame you get a perfectly balanced mountain bike that doesn't compromise handling for electric power.

These bikes are able to ride the same trails as their non-motorized counterparts. Black Diamond? No problem. Although the motor may seem exposed to bashes from rocks, the durable casing and bash guards - along with extra high clearance afforded by the full suspension geometry - make a perfectly capable housing for all that electric motor power. If you really want to get into detail, all of Haibike's innovative technologies are showcased here on Haibike's website.

So, why would you choose Haibike?

- You want to make it way easier to access trails at the top of long hills.
- You'd like a bike with enough torque to climb nearly anything.
- You're really into the idea of a silent electric motor.
- You want something that you can actually have fun with.
- You need to get away from the city for a little while."

Haibike Xduro Trekking RX – for the Urban Mountain

This review reproduced with permission from NYCeWheels – New York's finest electric bike store.

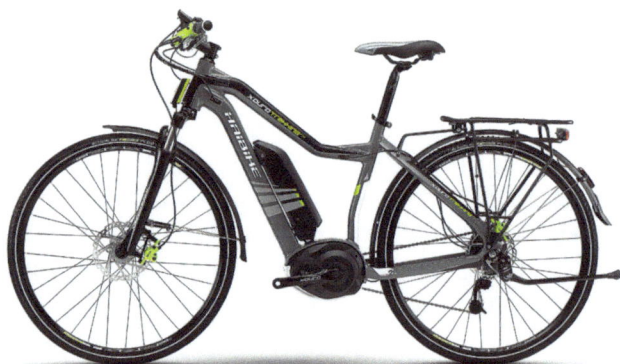

"Have you been looking for the ultimate bike to ride to work every day? Meet the Xduro Trekking RX - a lean mean commuting stallion! Torque and speed are equally important for commuters and you get plenty of both thanks to Haibike's Bosch Performance Center drive motor. Plus, the Xduro Trekking comes fully loaded with racks, fenders, lights and even a USB plug in the console so you can keep your phone charged!

Xduro Trekking RX features:

1. Bosch Center drive Performance system with a USB phone charger built in to console
2. Removable battery so you can charge your bike while you're at work
3. Great for light trails too!

The Bosch Center drive motor works right through the normal bicycle gears – just like you when you pedal. That makes it especially efficient on long hill climbs, repeated starts and stops, and over long distances with varied terrain. By working through the gears the motor of the Trekking RX can always operate in its most efficient range of RPMs – much like gears on a car – and deliver optimum performance to you as the rider.

For all your commuting needs, the Xduro Trekking is there, leaving you with no more excuses; save some money and leave your car at home!

IF Reach Folding Bike Review

This review reproduced with permission from NYCeWheels – New York's finest electric bike store. This review was written by Miles Schneider.

Dirt Bike Meets Road Racer

Once unfolded, it is hard not to notice the IF Reach's striking profile. It looks like a cross between a jacked-up dirt bike and sleek road racer – and that is more or less exactly what it is. Its lean frame and thin, road-gripping wheels make it clear that this is a bike built for speed, but the reinforced frame and dual-suspension give the Reach the ability to tear through whatever it runs into.

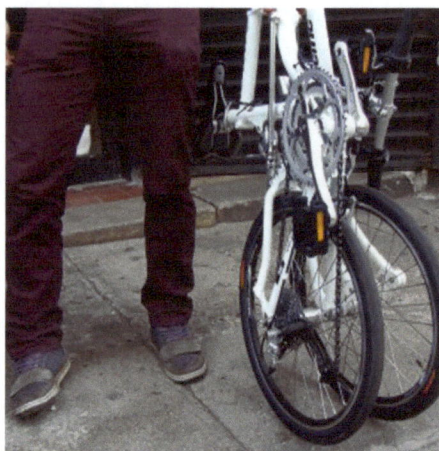

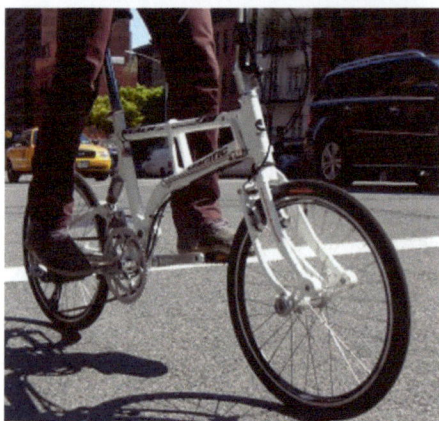

Now, you may be asking why a bike that is engineered for speed on concrete roads would feature front and rear shock absorbers. After all, shocks make a bike ride more cushy, but tend to slow you down since they abscond with some of the energy that gets put into pedaling. Pacific Cycles did their homework on this one, however. The shocks are extremely rigid, which means that don't seem to slow down the bike at all, but they do neutralize the vast majority of the instability and bumpiness associated with riding on 20-inch wheels. The result is a bike that can fold to a very compact size, but rides as convincingly like a full-size as any.

In fact, after riding nearly 20 miles on this bike, I am certain that I have never ridden a bike of any size with as impressive a combination of smoothness and speed. The sturdiness of the chassis also makes me eager to hook a trailer to this bike and see how it fares with a bit of cargo. After all, Pacific Cycles manufactures a variant on the IF Reach which features an electric motor and heavy battery, so it is clearly a frame that can take some stress. With any touring bike, smoothness, sturdiness, and speed are the three criteria to live and die by – you don't want anything so sluggish and heavy that it will slow you down, nor a bike that is so rigid that your arms will be numb from road vibration halfway through a day of riding. And of course, you need a frame that won't break under the combined weight of you and your camping gear. I have a sneaking suspicion that the IF Reach is the perfect combination of all these traits. It is certainly a tough, speedy bike, and I would love spending long days in its saddle exploring Oregon, New York, and beyond.

Kalkhoff Electric Bikes

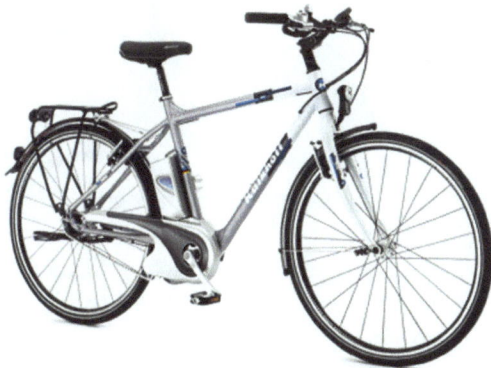

No review of electric bikes would be complete without a solid mention of the Kalkhoff. One day I hope to own one. Most people agree that the best drive system for an electric bike is the crank drive. Kalkhoff's crank drive is German engineered genius, their new Impulse crank drive system. It is said to be better than the excellent crank drives put out by Panasonic, Bosch and Yamaha.

Kalkhoff bikes are excellent quality and well equipped. These bikes have big batteries and efficient motors, giving them a range of almost 60 miles – which is very impressive in the electric bike world. It is also rumored that Kalkhoff are currently working on even sportier, faster, more powerful models that will be able to achieve up to 25 mph.

Kalkhoff also sells a cheaper model called the Groove, but it's just a collection of bits from China – not the beautiful fusion of German and Japanese engineering found in the rest of their range.

Kettler Twin Bikes

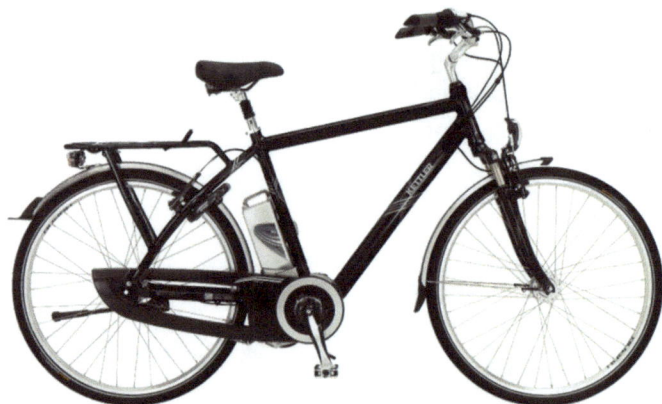

The Kettler Twin bikes are manufactured in Germany, and are really good quality. They use a Panasonic bottom-bracket 250-watt motor, and are very efficient. (Bear in mind that Panasonic was one of the pioneers in electric bike engines, so do not be fooled by the relatively small size of the engine – we are talking quality here.) They are available in a top tube or a step-through frame, and offer the option to get a basic LED display, or a multi-function LCD screen with better lights, and a Shimano Nexus

8-speed internal hub. The bikes come with a rack, fenders, and comfortable upright handlebars. Anyone from 5'0" to 6'5" can ride this bike, and the Lithium battery can reach over 30 miles per charge. This is a good one!

Kettler Twin Review

This review reproduced with permission from NYCeWheels – New York's finest electric bike store This review written by Seth.

With front suspension and a shock absorber in the seat post, the Kettler Twin electric bike provides a smooth and comfortable ride in even the harshest of conditions. The bike swallows up cracked pavement and uneven surfaces, allowing you to keep a steady pace at whatever speed you're traveling. The chewed up sections of pavement in the Lower East Side were no match for the plush suspension and relaxed feel of the Kettler ebike.

The Kettler Twin electric bike includes a built in rear rack that lets you attach a bag to carry your laptop to work, or blanket and some food if you're heading to the park for a picnic. A simple, spring-loaded clasp can hold a jacket or rain coat for days when you don't have a bag.

With the eight speed internal hub you'll have plenty of options for all sorts of riding. For long flat stretches of road or bike path, the higher gears will move you right along. At speed, the Kettler Twin electric bike feels solid and secure. When you head to the hills, the lower selection of gears allow the Kettler Twin electric bike to climb with ease.

The neat thing about the Kettler Twin electric bike is that it will let you do the work (pedaling!) if you want. When you're cruising along and spinning the pedals, the electric motor – which is wrapped around the crank set - will switch off and let you do the work. As you get stronger the bike will simply let you do more of the work!

But when you're unable to get the pedals spinning, the electric motor kicks in and helps move you along. Unlike other electric bikes that zip you along at the push of a button – you actually have to pedal on the Kettler Twin electric bike to get moving! This makes it more efficient and gives more of a feeling of riding a normal bicycle.

When you arrive at your destination, the Kettler Twin electric bike has a built in rear-wheel lock. The key stays in the lock until you clamp it around the wheel, then you can remove it. Its a good idea to use a bike lock to secure the bike to a stationary object if you leave it when going into a store or a cup of coffee, but the built in lock is a nice touch.

I was able to zip around New York City on the Kettler Twin for quite a while on just 3/5th of a charge. That was about 16 miles of biking around and even riding over the Williamsburg Bridge. I'm sure the more miles you ride, and the more you carry, the distance you can travel on one charge might be affected, but for a day of general riding around town I'm sure the Kettler Twin electric bike will be fine.

If you're new to cycling and are intimidated by hills, or the thought of riding more than a few miles, the Kettler Twin electric bike may be a great choice for you. Even if you're an experienced cyclist but just want a less strenuous ride over longer distances, this electric bike is great!

Montague Paratrooper Folding Mountain Bike Review

This review reproduced with permission from NYCeWheels – New York's finest electric bike store.

When I headed out on my first ride on the Montague Paratrooper I was unsure what to expect. I had seen a few of Montague's older videos of guys in camouflage riding the folding mountain bike through rivers and dirt trails and what not but that didn't really give me a good impression of what it's like.

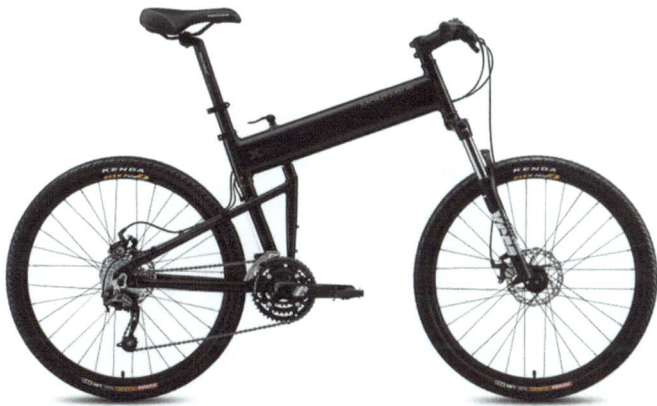

I'm not much of a mountain biker. I don't do downhill trails, dirt jumps, or anything too extreme. I do hit the occasional dirt road or run across a street full of pot holes though and I figured that the front suspension and sturdy frame design of the Paratrooper bike would lend itself to this sort of riding. On my very first ride I got a chance to try out each of these situations, plus I could take it on a ride through the NYC Subway system and test the folded size of the bike.

How does the Montague Paratrooper fold up?

I took the opportunity to fold my Montague Paratrooper several times before taking it out on the first ride. Compared to some other folding bicycle designs it doesn't fold up as small and it doesn't really stand up when folded. Then again, those small folding bicycles don't ride nearly as nice as the Paratrooper. Having large wheels is a positive and negative characteristic at the same time. On the one hand you have the positive characteristics of a smooth ride and nice handling and on the other hand you have the negative of not being as small when folded. If you have a bit more space for storage and you want to feel like you're riding a regular bicycle while riding your folding bike then you would prefer the Paratrooper.

Montague Paratrooper frame design and ride quality

The first think I noticed when I jumped on the Paratrooper folding bicycle was just how sturdy the frame felt. It was very stable when pedaling hard and tracked straight and true when flying down some of the hills around New York City. The disc brakes brought me to a satisfyingly quick stop each and every time I needed to slow my progress through the city streets. I love disc brakes by the way, they automatically push any bike that has them up a few notches in my mind.

Part of what makes the Montague Paratrooper such a stable bicycle is the super sturdy frame design. Unlike most folding bicycles which put a hinge right in the middle of the main tube the Paratrooper design swivels the frame around the seat post. This distributes the stress of your weight and pedaling force over a much larger area and prevents the frame from flexing each time you press on the pedals. Whenever the frame flexes you lose power and waste energy. The inflexibility of a bicycle frame is what makes it feel sturdy and confident – the less flex the better.

Paratrooper bike folded size

When folded up the Paratrooper bike does fit into some much smaller spaces than it's non-folding mountain bike cousins. For example, the Paratrooper bike can fit into the trunk of your car whereas a normal bicycle would have to go on a bike rack. The same applies for a boat, an RV, a plane, or any other short-on-space type situation.

Summary of my Paratrooper bike review

All in all I'd say the Paratrooper bikes – and Montague mountain bikes in general – have the best ride quality of any folding bicycle. They don't fold up super small but when folded they're already half the size of regular bikes. That makes all the difference for convenient storage and transport.

If you value ride quality over the size of the fold then you'll prefer the Montague Paratrooper over some of the other more compact folding bicycles.

Optibikes

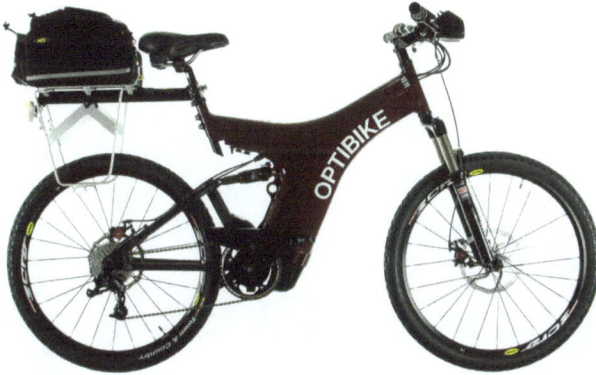

Optibikes are made in Boulder Colorado, and their web site claims they are the world's highest performing electric bikes. The *New York Times* referred to them as the Ferrari of electric bikes – and quite frankly, their price tag is reminiscent of a Ferrari too.

Run by Jim Turner, this company really does seem to be committed to building high quality electric bikes, and to be on the cutting edge of new electric bike development. Definitely worth checking out if you can afford the high prices – several thousand dollars, which is definitely on the very high end of prices.

The Optibike R Series is a mountain bike and looks the most like a real bike. They also offer the Optibike Helia, which is lighter and designed for women and comes in various colors including pink. These bikes are available with a 14 speed Rohloff Speedhub for ultra low maintenance, higher top speeds, and increased hill-climbing performance. And they are silent!

The Optibike is so reliable and handles so well that it is used by professional athletes as a pace bike at the Boulder Velodrome.

Finally, Optibike lets you have your bike custom-painted by two artists who also decorate Harley Davidsons. The results are impressive, to say the least – unique, artistic and eye-catching. These are not cheap bikes, but if I won the lottery, I'd probably buy one right away!

Pedal Easy Bike Review

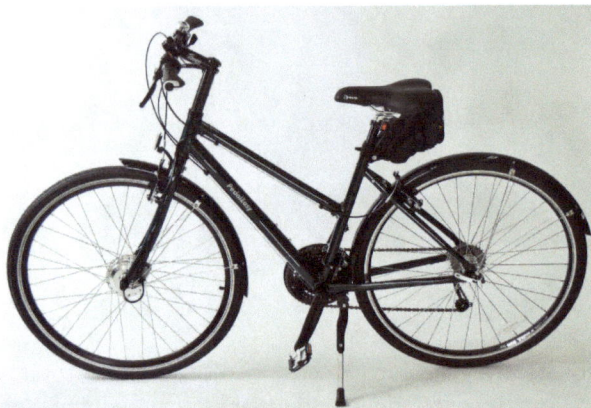

Ron Wensel is a Canadian engineer who has spent years testing and developing bike frames, batteries and motors, and has successfully developed a range of hand-assembled, lightweight, strong, easy-to-ride commuter electric bikes at an affordable price (around $1,500). I test rode one of his Pedal Easy bikes for a few months, and believe that he has done an excellent job.

Ron has always been a cyclist, but a series of heart attacks almost ended his cycling days. He was warned by his doctor that he had to keep his heart rate low. Instead of giving up cycling, Ron used his decades of engineering experience to develop a range of lightweight, long-range electric bikes. He pairs these lightweight bikes with small, high-efficiency batteries and discreet but powerful motors. These are not just any old batteries and motors. Ron described to me how he put all of the components through their paces, testing and dissecting them (literally) until he was sure he had top-rate components.

Pedal Easy Electric Bikes Look Like Regular Bikes

The first thing I noticed about my test bike is that it did not look like an electric bike. The battery is concealed in a saddlebag. The rear hub motor is so small and discreet that most people simply would not realize this is an electric bike.

I saw one of my fellow bike commuters in our bike parking the first time I rode it, and he said, "Oh, you're not on an electric bike" (because usually I do my long work commute on an electric bike). Now bear in mind that this guy is a serious cyclist, and he knows bikes. I said, "Actually it IS an electric bike," and he was quite shocked. I pointed out the engine in the almost-normal looking rear wheel hub and the battery hidden in the saddlebag. He said, "Wow, that's really discreet." He was even more impressed when I told him the price. And impressed again when I invited him to lift it up and see how light it was. With battery, the bike weighs in at just 28 pounds.

I can lift this bike onto my bike rack as easily as any regular bike. The Pedal Easy bike is a cinch to lift onto our Thule bike rack.

The Pedal Easy Electric Bike is Versatile

The great thing about these bikes is that you can pedal them like regular bikes when you don't need the electric assist. Ron tells me that some people have bought his bikes to use as regular bikes, because each one is a light, well-specced, extremely strong aluminium bike, well worth it's $1,500 price sticker, even if you don't need the engine.

What it Feels like to ride a Pedal Easy Electric Bike

The basic feeling you get on a Pedal Easy bike is SPORTY. You feel like you are on a high performance bike, cycling along with the strength of an Olympian.

I used the Pedal Easy to bike to work. I have a 22 km commute, with extreme and intermediate hills for the first 4 km. The bike I tested had only 3 speeds (there are other models with many more gears). Even so, the hills were pretty much a breeze. The bike weighs about 28 pounds, and I weigh about 170 pounds, for a grand total of around 200 pounds. So it's no mean feat to get us up very steep hills.

> I am happy to report that getting up steep hills is easy with a Pedal Easy electric bike.

The bike works entirely on a throttle basis. The throttle turns away from you, which took me a while to get used to (I have ridden motor cycles, which have throttles that turn the other way). I have to say that I love the throttle action. It's just so easy to pull off from a stop sign without putting pressure on my knees. And it's so much fun to use the throttle to manoeuvre through obstacles. It's very responsive and well calibrated, so you have a lot of manoeuvring ability. More so than on a regular bike, definitely.

The most fun part is simply zooming along without having to pedal at all. It's a great alternative for days when my knees are hurting. It even made me think about buying a motorcycle again, but I won't do that.

Pedal Easy Bikes Help you to Get Fit

A really good thing about the Pedal Easy is that you have to actually use the throttle for the engine to work. This is different from a Pedelec-type electric bike, where the engine kicks in as soon as you start pedalling, and is always there, matching your power output. This is good because you have to consciously engage the engine, so I find that very often I simply don't use the engine. I pretty much use the throttle when I need it, which means that I do a lot of regular cycling on the Pedal Easy. In fact, I substantially increased my fitness level while using it. Without it, I don't think I would have been fit enough to do the 30 kilometre MS Bike Tour recently.

I never thought I would ever be able to regularly tackle my difficult commute on a regular bike, but thanks to a couple of months of using the Pedal Easy, I have become so fit that I have now started doing this tough commute on a regular bike. I am very proud of this. It's one heck of a commute, and I could not have done it without months of getting fitter on a Pedal Easy electric bike.

This is what I love about electric bikes. You can use them to get fitter, you can use them on days when you are exhausted, or when your knees are hurting. You can use them to get over impossible hills. They take the angst out of long commutes, and flatten out really daunting hills. And of course, you can just plain have a whole lot of fun on them.

You can also use these electric bikes to lose weight, as I write about here.

Specs of the Pedal Easy Bikes

Pedal Easy bikes are nicely specced with reasonably high end Shimano components. They also come with good, practical wrap around fenders – essential for any bike commuter. And they look good!

The lightweight 320 W.h lithium-ion battery gets me about 35 km when I use it very heavily – basically, all the time. Charging takes a few hours. I recommend carrying a spare battery. That way, you always have a backup.

The engine is situated in the front hub. With the battery in the saddlebag, the balance of the bike is excellent.

Here are the complete specs of the 3 speed Pedal Easy Electric Bike:
- Frame & fork material: Double butted, 6061 aluminum, heat treated to T6
- Gearing: Shimano Nexus 3 speed
- Shifter: Shimano Revo-shifter
- Front/rear chain ring ratio: 48/18
- Tires: Kenda Kwest 700 x 35c touring/commuting
- Ergonomic handlebar grips
- Motor: 36 V, 350 W output power planetary-geared front hub
- Battery: Lithium-ion (Panasonic's latest NCR chemistry), 320 W.h capacity

- E-bike weight with battery, 16 kg (35 lbs)
- Cycle Analyst power meter and bio-responsive control system optional
- Styles: Standard (diamond-shaped) & step-through (sloped top bar)
- Sizes: 54 cm (standard frame), 45 cm (step-through)

Bottom Line on the Pedal Easy Electric Bike

I recommend Pedal Easy electric bikes to anyone who wants a great bike with plenty of electric assist available with just a flip of the wrist. They are excellent for commuting, and would also be an excellent choice for long bike tours. Pedal Easy also offers a range of Cycle Analyst power meters for precise display of e-bike parameter. They have some of the most cutting edge technology available in the world of electric bikes.

Sanyo Eneloop Electric Bike Review

This review reproduced with permission from NYCeWheels – New York's finest electric bike store.

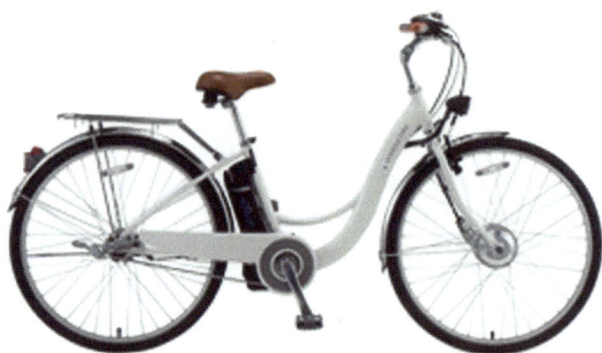

"The Sanyo Eneloop electric bike is super fun to ride, perfect for everyday commuters and recreational riders alike. It feels and handles like a regular bike and is even light enough to pedal with no battery power at all. Billed as a synergetic electric hybrid bicycle, the Eneloop uses the latest in regenerative braking and battery technology to combine your pedal power with an electric pedal assist.

Sanyo has been leading the electric battery industry for years. You can find there batteries in many popular electric bicycles, but this is the first fully-Sanyo electric bike. This bike is packed with awesome new technology that sets it apart from the thousands of electric bikes on the market.

Getting acquainted with the Sanyo Eneloop electric bike

Before we get into some of the more technical aspects of the Sanyo Eneloop electric bike. Let's check out some of the things that make it just plain cool! I look for features that make a bike useful and simple. I don't like complicated procedures or useless features. The Sanyo rates high for style and looks, and as it turns out, it its very easy to use too.

Battery

Installation and removal of the battery is a quick 2 step process. To install it you simply face the handle towards the rear wheel and rotate it into place. A nice solid click confirms a secure connection. The battery is now locked in place and safe to ride with. To remove it, insert and turn the key, then pull the battery towards you. It comes out effortlessly, with no resistance.

Controller

With the battery in place, we turn our attention to the controller. The controller on the Sanyo Eneloop electric bike may appear simple, with only three buttons, but don't be fooled. This easy to understand design puts all the information you need right under your nose. It has three buttons: on/off, mode, and lights on/off. The amount of charge remaining in the battery is indicated by three red LEDs above the on/off button. When fully charged there are three solid LEDs. You know it's time to recharge when the right hand LED blinks fast. There are three modes: auto, standard, and power-up. With auto mode the controller reads the force you are pedaling with and adjust power output accordingly up to a 1:2 ratio. On standard mode the motor will always assist pedaling with a 1:1 power ratio (putting in as much power as you do). Power-up mode assist pedaling at a 1:2 ration (twice as much motor power per pedal power).

Speeds

A three speed internal gear hub and twist style handlebar shifter make this one easy to ride bike. Shifting between the gears is a simple twist of the wrist. The gearing is similar to those classic 3 speed cruisers that are so much fun to ride. You have a gear for starting up and steep hills, one for going a little bit up-hill, and one for cruising and speed. That's all you need for most practical purposes, and it keeps things simple.

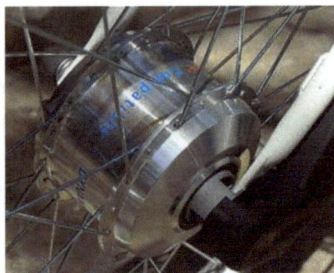

Lights

The lights on a Sanyo Eneloop electric bicycle are wired directly into the battery. No more need to spend extra money on expensive replacement batteries for the lights! They will even remain illuminated up to 15 minutes after pedal assistance is no longer available. When braking, the rear light will blink rapidly, regardless of whether the lights are on or off. Such ample lighting makes the Sanyo Eneloop electric bike very visible on crowded streets and dark roads.

Riding Position

With an adjustable handlebar stem and seat post this bike will fit most riders of an average height. I am over six foot and I felt a bit cramped when testing it, so taller riders should try the Eneloop for themselves to see if they feel comfortable before buying.

Some Extras

Every Sanyo Eneloop electric bicycle comes with a large durable rear rack and a sturdy rear wheel mounted kick stand. It's too bad the guys at Sanyo didn't think to make the rear rack removable. You could easily put some coals under it and it would be a perfect hibachi grill. Think of the picnics you could have!

Now that we've gotten to know the basic features of the Sanyo Eneloop electric bike lets dive right into what makes Sanyo electric bike one of the best electric bicycles

An ultra light, ultra long lasting battery

A high-performance lithium-ion battery is at the heart of the Sanyo Eneloop electric bike. Lithium-ion batteries are lighter and longer lasting that older battery technologies. They also charge faster and last longer. What more could you want? The battery in the Sanyo Eneloop weighs about 3.3 lbs, compare that to average electric bike batteries that weigh 7 to 10 lbs. Under ideal conditions it takes about 3 hours and 30 minutes to fully charge the battery. A full charge can power you for up to 40 miles, depending on riding conditions. That's enough to get you to and from most local destinations without recharging. When properly used these batteries will last for about 300 to 500 charge/discharge cycles, or about a year and a half. Overcharging and improper storage can reduce their life span. The Sanyo Eneloop electric bike certainly has the most advanced battery technology of any electric bicycle.

Take care of your battery, don't leave it in a corner to sulk. Batteries need love too you know! Long periods of neglect will make them cranky and inefficient. If you plan on storing your battery, take proper care of it so you don't wind up with a really expensive useless brick. Batteries naturally self-discharge over time, so you should check their charge about once a month and charge for an hour if they go below 25% charge. The battery should be stored in a cool place, not more than 50% charged. A fully charged battery can be dangerous and should be run down before storage. If the battery is left for a long time without charging it can become over discharged and lose its ability to fully charge. Storing the battery won't necessarily increase the usable life of the battery, proper storage will keep the battery in good working order when it is not being used.

Sanyo Eneloop electric bike dynamotor works wonders

The key to the Eneloop electric bike's pedal assistance is it's front hub Dyna-motor. The Dyna-motor is a dual function front hub motor and dynamo generator (hence dyna-motor!) which is both powered by the battery and recharges it. Gently applying the rear brake on a downhill slope starts an electric braking process within the dyna-motor which uses the bike's momentum to charge the battery. Don't try to go too fast thinking you are charging the battery faster, the battery will not recharge if the bike is traveling over 15 mph.

Leave other electric bikes behind!

The Sanyo Eneloop electric bike has a great battery and a super light frame, making it a front runner in the long distance electric bike market. Regenerative braking in combination with intelligent pedal assistance increases its range over other electric bikes. In auto mode, using regenerative braking on downhills, the Sanyo Eneloop electric bicycle can go for 32 to 40 miles with out stopping. On a flat road you can get 13 to 16 miles on power-up, 13 to 23 miles on standard, and 22 to 26 miles on auto.

And when your battery finally runs out, you can still make it home without too much trouble thanks to the bike's light frame. I rode it for a few miles with no pedal assist and found it to perform about as well the average 3 speed cruiser.

Intelligent power assistance:

How did they make the acceleration and pedal assistance on this electric bike so smooth and responsive? The secret to the power assistance on a Sanyo Eneloop electric bike is the crank sensor, located within the bottom bracket of the bike. The crank sensor reads how much pressure, or torque, you put into the pedals. The controller then calculates a proportional pedal assistance according to what mode it is set to. Take standard mode for example. When you start pedaling the crank sensor reads your pedal force and adds exactly the same amount of motor assistance, doubling your overall power on the bike. This is a 1:1 ratio of pedal to motor power. As you pass 6.2 mph the maximum ratio of pedal power to motor power decreases gradually. When you pass 15 mph the motor no longer assists pedaling. As soon as you stop pedaling or apply the rear brake the pedal assist stops. This smooth and responsive pedal assistance makes riding the Sanyo Eneloop electric bicycle feel more like riding a regular bike.

To sum it all up, the Sanyo Eneloop electric bike is totally awesome.

The Sanyo Eneloop electric bicycle really surprised me with how much it felt like riding a regular 3 speed bike. With 3 modes of smooth intelligent power assistance you can feel the additional power without feeling out of control. A high-performance lithium-ion battery gives it the range for longer rides and commutes, and saves you several extra pounds of weight over older battery technologies. Relatively short charging time gets you back on the road again without having to charge overnight. All in all, I'd say that the Sanyo Eneloop electric bicycle is far superior to most electric bikes, it can go farther and last longer. It is definitely one amazing electric bike.

Schwinn Electric Bikes

Schwinn has a checkered career with regular bikes – some are stellar, some are not – and their enterprising foray into electric bikes seems to be similarly checkered. They are known to have made some mistakes, yet at the same time their Tailwind model is much loved by many collectors. To make the matter all the more confusing, it's not possible to find any information about their electric bikes on their own web site. Searches on the words "electric," "ebikes" and "Tailwind" brings up "no results found." It seems that Schwinn doesn't actually want to sell these bikes. Nonetheless, I have tried to find out what I can about them.

Unsurprisingly, I have read very mixed reviews on the Tailwind, but most of them are glowing – a strong, sturdy urban bike with all the necessaries, 8 gears that are said to be just right, and an incredibly fast battery recharge (around 30 minutes). Of course, if you want to buy one, you would somehow have to find it, and Schwinn's website is not going to help you.

Strida 5.0 Review

This review reproduced with permission from NYCeWheels – New York's finest electric bike store.

I'm coming upon my 1 year anniversary with my Strida 5.0 folding bike, and I chose to mark the occasion by completing a sopping wet five-borough bike tour. The Strida certainly sparked lots of chatter along the route, with at least two individuals asking whether I had built the bike myself, which I imagine is because of the bike's clearly minimalist design. So you're probably wondering, what's it like doing 42 miles on the Strida? The answer: Peachy! In contrast to NyceWheel's own caution for riding 100 miles on the Strida, I actually haven't found the bike's riding position uncomfortable – even over a 42 mile stretch. That said, I definitely wouldn't ride for too long while wearing any sort of backpack/messenger bag; I encountered some

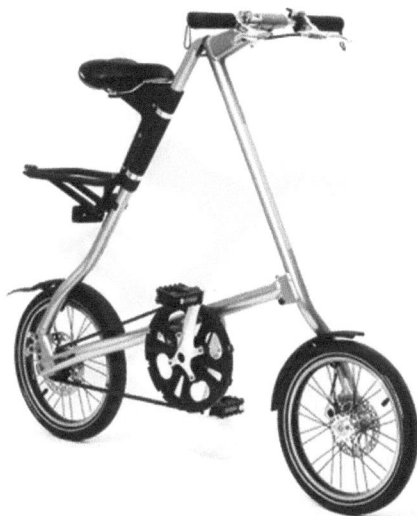

much dreaded numbness during a mere 5 mile trip while wearing my Camelbak. Due to the upright riding position, it's really hard to carry anything on your back.

During these past months, I've commuted roughly 60 miles/week during every month except January. I've found several worthwhile accessories along the way, though none that are specifically made for the Strida. I use NiteRider MiNewt X2 dual beam headlights on the front end, an Arkel Tail Rider pannier on the bike's rear rack and a Lightman xenon strobe on each side of the lower portion of the rear rack so I can be seen by perpendicular traffic. I added Strida's after-market kickstand to the bike, but had to remove it within a short time.

Not only did the kickstand interfere with the fold, but it also seemed to weigh down the belt-tension bolt to which it was anchored. I'm guessing a mechanic could have found a way to eliminate the problem, but it seemed kind of silly that one would need to hire a mechanic to install an after-market kickstand (which is why I didn't hire one). The best upgrade I've made is the switch to Schwalbe's Big Apple tires. The ride is infinitely more stable and, quite frankly, secure as a result of this change.

The Big Apple's truly approximate an elastometer-grade suspension fork, and I can't recommend this upgrade enough. Unfortunately, this change has come at a cost: the bike's ability to be wheeled along while folded is significantly compromised. The Big Apple tires are much thicker, requiring that several washers be inserted behind each wheel's magnetic connections in order to accommodate the increased width. While the added washers allow the bike to fold completely, the connection is definitely weaker, and the bike's folded halves unclip as soon as I begin to roll the Strida. In short, one of the bike's best features – its ability to roll while folded – seems to be mutually exclusive with a very valuable upgrade, namely the switch to Schwalbe's Big Apple tires. I'm not willing to give up the Big Apples, but I do miss the added portability and will continue to search for a workaround.

Since purchasing the Strida, I have become a full-time bike commuter. I ride in all conditions except ice and snow, and, because I so love riding the Strida, I'm always looking for new bike-commuting opportunities throughout the week and weekends. The Strida's definitely been a great commuting platform, and, as a non-profit worker who demands a large return on any cycling investments, it's absolutely exceeded my expectations.

Stromer Review

This review reproduced with permission from NYCeWheels – New York's finest electric bike store.

Stromer ST1 Platinum Bike shops see electric bicycles a little differently than their customers do. We work with the distributor or manufacturer directly – developing a relationship that can either make us excited to sell every bike or make us wonder whether we'll still carry them next year. As a dealer looking to carry an electric bike we

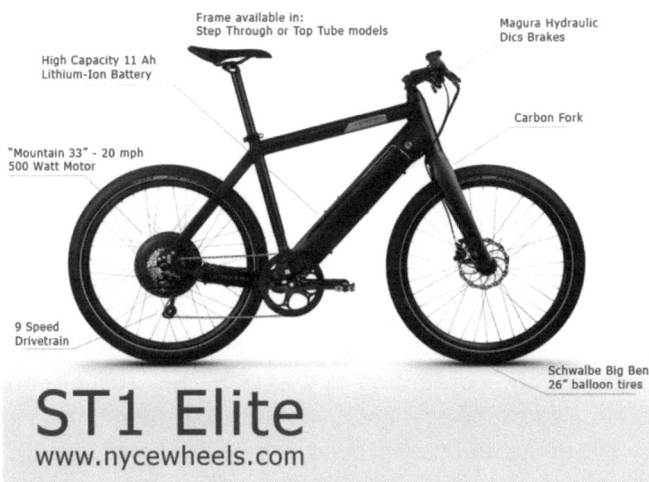

Frame available in:
Step Through or Top Tube models

Magura Hydraulic
Dics Brakes

High Capacity 11 Ah
Lithium-Ion Battery

Carbon Fork

"Mountain 33" - 20 mph
500 Watt Motor

9 Speed
Drivetrain

Schwalbe Big Ben
26" balloon tires

ST1 Elite
www.nycewheels.com

want all the same stuff you might as a customer – looks that could kill, performance that is felt while riding rather than read in a press release, good quality workmanship, and good support.

My work with Stromer BMC selling the ST1 Elite and ST1 Platinum has been some of the most fun I've had at NYCeWheels in the last 3 years. To put that in perspective, let's flash back to when I just started here, way back in 2010 ... (cue Twilight Zone music).

At the time we had a full line of electric bikes but they were all pretty basic looking, had clunky controls attached to the handlebar and very basic interface. More than that though, they lacked a certain refinement found on regular bicycles.

Skip ahead to 2011 when we got our first Stromer Sport model on the sales floor. This bike out shone everything else in the shop. It looked cooler, worked better, and rode nicer than any other bike we carried. I remember that first ride – I was blown away by how much like a regular bicycle it looked. I loved the frame mounted battery and mountain bike looks. I loved the clearly readable display that didn't look like an Atari strapped to the handlebar. In fact, I still like that bike. I rode it home and back the other day and it still kicks butt.

Flash forward to now, we've had the Stromer ST1 for about a year and I feel electric bicycles are finally starting to attain the sort of beautifully sculpted, well balanced look found in the regular bicycle world. Just like my first experience with the Stromer Sport – my first encounter with the ST1 was a moment of true excitement. Here is a bicycle I can get behind. Here is a bicycle I'm excited to sell!

Look at that carbon fork! You see how it accents the shape and stance of the bike? Don't you love the feeling of beefy speed that it adds to the front end? Stromer dared to challenge the convention of always putting suspension forks on electric bikes – heck, we even told them it was a risk – but in the end they proved to be on the leading edge of something amazing. Of course, they still offer suspension models for folks who'll be on and off dirt trails a whole bunch but for those of you who ride the pavement most often the carbon fork is really where it's at.

I'm getting a little carried away with looks, you can already judge those for yourself. Let's get back to what I see as a dealer, rather than a customer.

Selling a bunch of bikes you get to know whether they're reliable or not. You also get to know whether the maker will jump to the line to help its customers or whether they'll blow things off and not take care of business. Stromer has performed incredibly well on both counts.

Any bike, no matter how perfect, can have a problem. What's critical is how the company deals with these problems. Everything is better and easier with a company that stands behind their product. Stromer has proved very capable of supporting their dealers and customers in tough situations by providing the knowledge and initiative necessary to get things done right and done quickly.

If you're thinking of getting an electric bicycle, I'd really recommend you look into a Stromer.

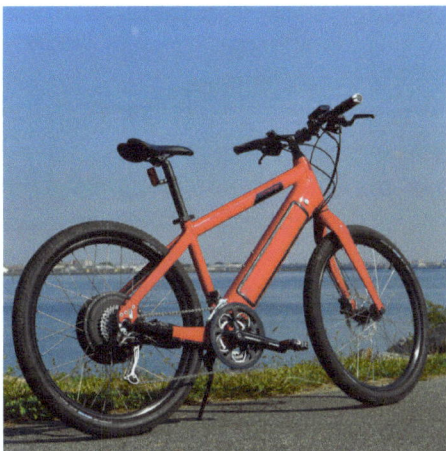

Another Stromer Review, this one from Turbo Bob

This review reproduced with permission from NYCeWheels — New York's finest electric bike store — and with permission from Turbo Bob, one of the greatest online electric bike reviewers. I highly recommend Bob's blog, which you can find at https://turbobobbicycleblog.wordpress.com/

I've ridden more than a few Stromer electric bikes, but this one I'm on now is the best ever. You may think the 'talk to me' red paint job is what's catching my fancy, yet it's so much more than that. Styled in pure European fashion, in reminds me of some classic motorbikes I rode and raced in my youth and some race versions I only dreamed of taking to the track.

As I pulled it from the shipping carton, I was in awe of its looks and features. It took the shortest time to get it up and running, with a quick blast around the neighborhood before setting the battery on the charger. As the battery filled with go juice, I poured over the bike to check all the settings and just soak-up what was to come. I even checked the owners manual to see how the display operates. Not something that everyone does, but worth the time and effort.

Finally ready to go, I hopped aboard for a long shake-down run. This Stromer Platinum didn't disappoint as the miles melted away. Even though it has plenty of gears, I spent most of my time in the upper ones, as the smooth power from the rear hub motor makes the lower ones less important to my riding style. Working between the four levels of assist, I was always happy with the acceleration and cruising speed it offered.

Stromer ST1: a pure experience

You can get the Stromer ST1 in a few different configurations. The Platinum has no throttle and the motor is motivated only with your pedaling. A very sensitive torque-sensing control system feels what you want and delivers right now. Unlike most E-bikes on the market, this type of control gives you the most pure of E-bike experiences. It is a bike rider's bike and makes most pale in comparison with the power and seamless smoothness it deals up.

The 2013 Stromer shares much with the older models I have ridden. The lithium battery is enclosed in the frame tube and has a nice mechanism that allows access to it. It can be charged in the bike or separate depending on your needs. It has a sporty seating position that is a middle ground between road bike and cruiser. It very much has the mountain bike look and I imagine it could be ridden just about anywhere.

This year's tires have a larger cross-section, something that I was glad to see. And of course they are name brand top-end tires that should give miles of service with a smile and no flats. The front fork is carbon fiber, yet with this flawless paint job it is hard to tell. The aluminum frame matches in that vibrant red. You can opt for other colors and a low-framed model as well. Check the Stromer ST1 NYCeWheels page for all your choices.

This Platinum has a little more get up and go than most E-bikes you might consider getting. Because it only can power-up while you are pedaling, the rules allow a few more mph than most. In fact without working up a major sweat it can pull 30 of those mph in no time at all. On top of the extra oomph, it also has a larger capacity battery to extend your rides even at the higher speeds. I normally keep the speed to under 20, but those power blasts are a 'blast'.

So the draw with this Stromer Platinum are many: great looks; top-end components; fine handling; long range; plenty of power; battery regeneration on the down-grades; super brakes; precise and smooth motor-assist control – and many more that you might have to find on your own.

When I say this bike has 'nothing you don't' need, I am overlooking the optional 'city kit'. A set of fenders and lights could round out the package for many. I always add some lights to any bike I ride. Yet the 'stripped' and 'racy' look of this bike might be the way you desire and need. It's up to you of course.

Go Stromer and go strong, Turbo Bob

Tern Verge X20 Review

This review reproduced with permission from NYCeWheels – New York's finest electric bike store. This one was written by Jody Brooks

This is a review of the 2012 Tern Verge X20 folding bicycle, one of 6 folding bicycles in the Verge line. Verge bikes are a set of folding bicycles focused on speed/performance with 20 inch wheels.

What initially distinguishes each Verge bike model is the number of gears, represented in their model numbers. In general, more gears means more options when climbing. Also, if the gear ratios are right, more gears also means more speed on the flats.

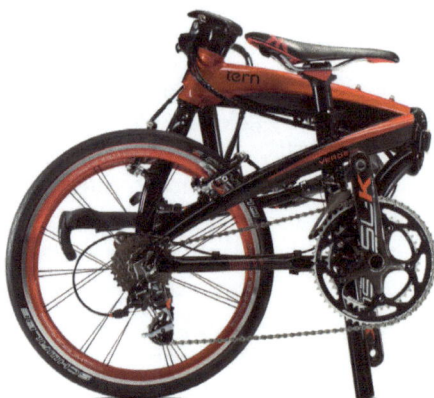

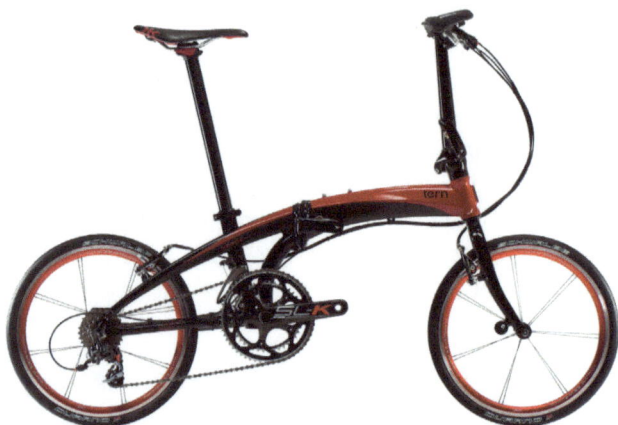

Each Tern Verge model is distinguished beyond its gear range with things like overall speed, internal shifting, overall weight, etc. The Verge X20 really stands out because it excels in not just one, but many, of these aspects.

As we'll see, the Verge X20 delivers high performance

The X20 is a folding bicycle with a minimum of compromises. Some may feel the X20 does this by compromising your bank balance. It is not a cheap folding bike. However, even on this score, the Verge X20 compares favorably to other high performance folding bikes on the market.

Components: Verge 20 Shifting

Initially, what stands out on the Verge X20 are the components: both for their performance pedigree and their aesthetic appeal. The SRAM Red shifting on the X20 includes the exact same set of SRAM front and rear derailleurs that provide the lightning fast, crystal clear, shifting found on many top of the line road bicycles.

The one obvious difference is in the shifters which are designed for a straight handlebar. Otherwise, you enjoy the same fantastic shifting on your folding bike as you would on any high end regular bicycle.

Components: Verge X20 Drivetrain

The Verge X20's bike bling continues with the FSA SL-K carbon crankset. Again, the same kind of crank set you find on many high end road bicycles. The only difference here is a pair of extra large front chain rings made custom for Tern. Instead of a standard 53/39 tooth count for the front chain ring, the Verge 20 ships with a 55/42 tooth count. This comes in handy later. If you've never seen it, check out some Verge X20 pictures.

With 20 different gears into which you can shift, the Tern X20 is second only to the Verge X30h for shifting options in the Verge line. That said, gears are only as good as the ratio.

Components: Tern X20 Gear Ratio

A chronic challenge for bikes with smaller wheels, like the Verge line of folding bikes, is increasing the gear ratio between the front and rear gears, respectively. This helps compensate for the higher rate of revolution with smaller wheels. This web page by Sheldon Brown provides a concise explanation of the issue.

Typically, the gear ratio issue gets resolved by reducing the rear gear tooth count, increasing the front gear tooth count, or doing the equivalent with proprietary gear systems set inside the rear hub.

For example, the Verge X30h invokes the latter option by way of the SRAM Dual Drive II internal hub shifting system. This has the effect of turning the Verge X30h's front chain ring from 53T to ~71T. This gives the Verge X30h top end gearing that rivals many road bikes. That is incredible.

Tern Verge X20: Extending the standard

Still, with anything proprietary or non-standard to the road bike world, service can sometimes be hard to come by. The Verge X20 overcomes proprietary gear shifting pitfalls while still delivering a nice top end gearing by extending the front end of a standard drivetrain. The rear cassette is the same you find on a standard road bike: 11/28 or 11/32 tooth range. The difference is simply that the front chainrings are slightly larger than what is normally found on a regular road bike.

This produces a lower top end gearing than you find on the Verge X30h and a few other folding bikes. However, the top end gearing is still respectable on the flats and downhill. I find I can sustain 30kph with a moderate cadence and 35kph by really winding out. I won't be winning any downhill road races but 30kph is slightly higher than the average speed on the flats that I achieve with my standard road bike so the Verge X20 rarely feels like a sacrifice. And again, down the road, maintenance of the X20 drivetrain should be stress-free thanks to standard and ubiquitous parts.

Weight! The Verge X20 weighs just 9.3 kg (20.5 lb). That makes it the lightest of the Verge series and the lightest folding bicycle Tern makes this year. In fact, it is one of the lightest folding bicycles on the market.

There are lighter folding bicycles with comparable components. Bikes like the Bike Friday PR Super Pro Red weigh in at 7.5 kg (16.5 lbs). However, it only supports riders of 86.36 kg (190 lb) while the Tern Verge X20 supports riders of 110 kg (243 lb). That's a huge difference to 200 pounders like me.

Stability! The weight specs reveal one of the great strengths of Terns in general and the Verge X20 in particular. So many folding bikes on the market have a feel that ranges from unstable to downright flimsy. This is not the case with Tern.

Descending! The Verge X20, like the rest of the line, feels really solid. My bike commute begins with a 300 meter descent in less than a mile of terrain. The Verge X20 performs this beautifully. I can't say it is as stable as my full size carbon road bike but it is still spectacular for such a small and light bike; not to mention, one that folds.

Climbing! The stability continues up hill as well. With such a steep climb home, I want every bit of my precious energy transferred to the wheels and that's how the Verge 20 feels. Although the frame geometry has a lot to do with it, the Verge X20 design has a minimal quality that eliminates unwanted flex and shift within the frame.

Verge X20 – Stable in hand, stable under foot

Terns avoid the telescoping handlebar stems found on other folding bikes. This removes one more part that could flex or shift when climbing. Instead, Terns use a simple, ingenious, handlebar clamp that pivots up and down. After several trips up my hill, the whole handlebar assembly still feels solid.

There's also a minimum of flex at the pedal thanks to the standard road bike carbon cranks and Tern's simple, yet strong, frame geometry. Don't forget to order some pedals with your bike, or plan on using a spare set you have lying around. Like any high end road bike, it doesn't come with pedals.

The Verge X20 climbs and descends beautifully. Except for really fast paced or high mile road rides, I can't see missing my road bike. This is more than I ever expected from any commuter bike or, much less, a folding bike.

Another factor in the feel of stability, is the fit of the Tern X20. Most people that ride my Verge X20 are astonished by how similar the saddle, pedal and handlebar placement feel to a regular bicycle. However, since I am 190.5 cm (6'3") tall with an extraordinarily long torso, the fit on the Verge X20 was initially a concern. Nevertheless, I was able to resolve this easily with a seat adjustment and a 3 cm riser handlebar. Regardless, mine is a unique case. I've since seen many six footers fit the stock configuration just fine.

As for legroom, there is plenty. Even for my large self, this was never an issue. I do have to max out the seat post height but it still feels stable and I feel fine. This is incredible for a folding bike that is so light.

Last but not least, the Verge X20 is one of the most beautiful folding bikes made. The Verge X20 has Tern's trademark frame, an elegant arch of hydroformed aluminum, coated with glossy black and deep metallic red paint.

The super thin red anodized 20 inch wheels top off the attractive components and frame to make a truly striking folding bike that turns heads wherever I go. I've heard more than one folding bike skeptic say the Verge X20 overcomes the aesthetic issues some have had with small wheeled folding bikes.

BTW: It Folds...Beautifully

With all the great features of the Verge X20, it is easy to forget that it folds: beautifully. Like most Terns bikes, and very few other folding bikes, the Verge X20 is super easy and quick to fold. In general, Terns fold into a simple N-shaped pattern, across a single plane. This makes the folding process very intuitive and/or the easiest to remember of any folding bike I have encountered.

The one minor weakness to the folding process is the locking mechanism. At each folding point, Tern clamps employ a tiny sliding button that locks the clamp. The innards of these locking buttons are made of plastic. They work great. However, they do snap off easily when the uninitiated tug on the hinge clamp before sliding the lock. Although these pins are easily replaced, these incidents make it unclear how much locking value these pins provide if they break so easily. Perhaps these locking pins would work better as metal.

Wrapping it up – Verge X20!

The Tern Verge X20 succeeds in being a folding bike that delivers a broad range of performance with very few compromises.

Some hardcore speed demons might object to the top end speed but few cyclists can sustain the Verge X20's top speed on the flats for very long anyway. What's more, no one will be wanting for gears when climbing. The low range is great and the SRAM Red shifting delivers the gears you need at the right time.

Some may take issue with the price of the Verge X20, which is the highest in the Verge series. However, no bike in the Verge series and very few folding bikes on the market have a comparable set of high end components. These components cost a lot no matter what bike on which they are mounted. In fact, the only other folding bike shipping with SRAM Red shifting components, the Bike Friday Super Pro Red, costs over twice as much as the Verge X20!

The combination of performance, speed, reliability, maintainability, and reasonable if not low pricing, will make this the right choice for many weekend road warriors who want or need a fast, folding, commuter.

Emotion BH Race Bike with Panasonic Mid-Drive Bike Motor

The BH Emotion is a Panasonic Electric Bike that looks like a handsome, sleek road bike. And it handles like a stiff, responsive road bike. However, it does have a secret: a crank drive electric assist bike motor concealed under a chain guard, powered by a lightweight Panasonic battery on the seat tube. The BH Emotion bike is powered by one of Panasonic's legendary mid-drive bike motors.

The Panasonic Electric Bike is a Pedelec, NOT a Motorbike

Just to get this out of the way first: this bike is for people who still want to get plenty of exercise. If you want something that will move without any effort, this bike is not for you. If you want to move fast and powerfully WITH effort, then this bike could work for you. The Emotion BH E9502 Race Bike does not have a throttle – it is a Pedelec, meaning that the power only kicks in when you pedal.

On this bike, the power kicks in IMMEDIATELY when you pedal.

Many bikes have a few seconds delay on the motor, for safety reasons, but that can make it really hard to pull off on an uphill. So I really prefer this option. The downside is you have to be careful how you rest your feet on the pedals when stopped – if you accidentally apply pressure, the bike can jerk forward.

About Panasonic mid-drive bike motors

The Panasonic bike motor was invented in the early 1990s, when Yamaha and Panasonic began building drive systems for pedal assist electric bicycles. The Panasonic bike motor has always been very reliable, but in the 25 years since it was invented, battery technology has improved in leaps and bounds. That means that bike riders now get to enjoy an incredibly powerful combo (what I like to call the Dynamic Duo) – the Panasonic bike motor and the Panasonic battery. That means we have more power and great range!

The Dynamic Duo is now offered on a whole range of excellent bikes, manufactured by great names such as Kalkhoff, Focus, Raleigh, KTM, Helkama, and BH Easy Motion (Emotion). The bike I have is from BH's Emotion range. BH is a bike manufacturer in Spain that has been turning out bikes for more than a hundred years. BH Bikes are regularly seen on the podium at international bike races.

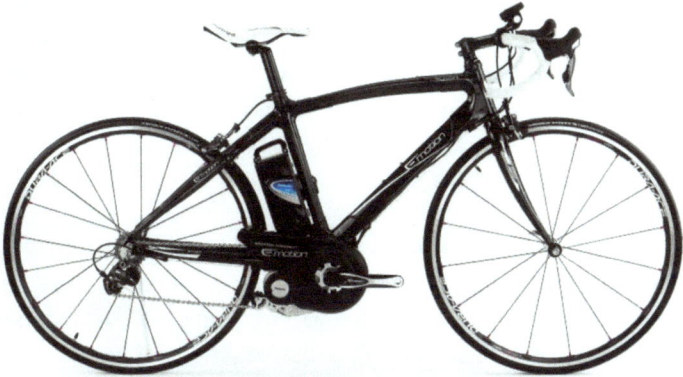

Electric Motor + Pedals + Gear System = Speed and Power on Your Panasonic Electric Bike

The key to the power and the grace of this Panasonic bike motor – the key thing that makes it an industry benchmark for performance and reliability – is the motor in the middle. Because the motor and battery are in the middle, near the crank drive, the motor draws powerfully on the mechanical advantage of the bike gears. This means that a relatively small bike motor is amplified, delivering efficient power. Power that I can I feel every time I ride my Emotion BH Race Bike up a hill and pass guys who are 20 years younger than me. Essentially, having the gears integrated with the crank drive motor means that you can keep the engine in its high RPMs by downshifting. When you downshift on a regular bike you can end up with almost no power, but that is NOT the case here.

The BH – Panasonic Electric Bike - Combo: Great Bike Maker Partners up with Great Motor Maker

The BH Emotion E9502 Race bike comprises a 250 W Panasonic engine and battery, mounted on a specially crafted BH Bike. BH has been making bikes for over a hundred years in Spain, and the quality shows. BH Emotion is their electric assist line, which is the result of partnering with Panasonic and Samsung. Emotion also manufactures the award-winning line of Neo mountain bikes, as well as road bikes and cross (hybrid) bikes. They claim to have the lightest electric road bike in the world, in their all-carbon road bike. My Panasonic electric bike, weighing in at a modest 37 pounds, is one of the world's lightest electric bikes.

This bike integrates a crank drive 250W Panasonic mid-drive motor with 10-speed Shimano 105 gears. If you've ever ridden a bike with Shimano 105 gears, you will know that they are smooth and impressive. The combination of the Panasonic mid-drive motor with Shimano 105 gears combines the best of all worlds, integrating the brilliance of a smooth geared system with the efficiency of an electric bike motor. The bike of course has a complete Shimano 105 set, so the brakes are also Shimano 105.

You control the motor via the console on the handle bars, which essentially has an On button, a choice of 3 levels of power, and an indicator to tell you how much power is left in your battery.

A lot of electric bike lovers might sneer at the very idea of a 250 W engine – to them I say, just TRY this Panasonic Electric Bike for hills AND speed!

Note that the number of gears is relatively low because the usual front cogs are replaced by the crank drive motor. So you don't have 10 x 2 or 3 – you just have 10. However, in my experience 10 speeds is more than enough on an electric bike.

A great thing about having the motor in the crank drive and the battery on the seat tube is that the bike is very well balanced, handling exactly like a regular bike.

A nice feature of this bike is that it is quite long. This means I never have to worry about boot-hitting-front-tire (even though I wear boots, not cycling shoes, when I ride). It also means there is plenty of space for your panniers, without ever having that disconcerting feeling when your heel hits a pannier.

Operation

The battery mount works with a key. You cannot take the battery off without turning the key. Once you turn the key, the battery slides off with the greatest of ease. Then you turn the key back to the mounting position and leave it that way. You take the battery and pop it neatly into the charger, which is a nice square unit that lies securely on the ground, plugged into a regular wall socket. A full charge takes about an hour. When you come back to the bike, the battery slides back in smoothly and easily with nice little click to tell you it is in place.

Then you get on the bike, press the On button, select from 3 levels of assistance, and off you go. You can also turn the assist on and off while you are moving, in case you want to increase your exercise. As soon as you start pedaling, the motor starts working.

Carbon forks

The BH E9502 Race Bike is an aluminum road bike with carbon forks. It is ideal for long commutes, and for those who like to go fast on their commutes. It's also ideal for cyclists like me who want to do long commutes without a car, but have limited time and less-than-perfect knees. Bear in mind though, that it is a stiff road bike, so you may find it tough on your elbows. There are no shocks to absorb the potholes.

Also, as it is so light, you can easily pedal it without assistance in the unlikely event you run out of battery charge. Once I ran out of battery charge. But I was zooming along so fast, that I did not actually notice until I came to an uphill! And even then, I was able to get up the hill without embarrassment. By contrast, on heavier electric bikes, when the power cuts out, it feels like someone slammed the brakes on.

The Panasonic motor is close to noiseless, and utilizes a proportional torque sensor to add power equivalent to how hard you are pedaling.

No Speed Limit!

A nice thing about these bikes is that it is really easy to override the ridiculous 32-km per hour limit that is imposed on many electric bikes. It's a very simple adjustment, which your dealer may be willing to make for you. This means that when you are zooming along at speed, you don't suddenly have the power cut out as you hit 32 km per hour. (When they start to put 60 km per hour limits on car engines, I MAY be ready to accept speed limits on bike engines.)

Panasonic 36 V Li-ion Battery

The battery is a Lithium-ion (Li-ion), 36 V (8 Ah). You can upgrade to a 48 V (9 or 12 Ah) for greater range, which I would recommend if you can afford it. However, I am doing just fine with a 36 V, and my commute is 20 miles round trip.

I love the lightweight Panasonic battery, with its easy-carry handle, which makes it easy for me to carry it up to my office and recharge it as I work. However, you most likely won't need to take it up to your office, as this setup has a range of at least 20 miles, even using the motor at full capacity (you can choose from an assistance level of 1, 2 or 3).

The battery has 3 lights on the console to tell you how much power remains, and then 5 lights on the battery itself, which gives you a more precise (but still very vague) indication. All you know is that you have between 1 and 20% of power left when one light is on. And to see the lights on the battery, you need to dismount and press the button on the battery.

I would like to see this system with a more precise battery meter on the console.

Warranties

The bikes, engines and batteries are warrantied for two years, and are of excellent quality. One downside is that an extra charger will cost you around $300, which compares unfavorably with a BionX charger at around $100.

BionX Batteries versus Panasonic Batteries

When I started riding this bike I used to travel 22 km to work using the bike motor at full power, doing a lot of huge hills. By the time I got to work I would be down to 1 bar out of 3, and I recharged before I biked home again. After riding it for a few months I am so much fitter that I can do the full 44 km round trip on one battery charge, and still have juice to spare.

All bike batteries deteriorate of course, and it is extremely hard to quantify, unless one keeps precise records for years, and I just don't do that kind of thing. It is my subjective impression that this battery initially lost quite a bit of charge (maybe 15%) quite quickly (6 months), but since then has levelled out and just seems to go on forever. Overall, I think it is even better than the BionX battery.

Looks and Performance of the Panasonic Electric Bike

This bike looks awesome! I often have guys on the street say to me: "What a beautiful bike!" I believe most of them don't realize it is an electric bike. I also have little boys looking at my bike with mouths hanging open, just saying "Wow!"

Make no mistake; this Panasonic Electric Bike is a handsome piece of machinery. I LOVE it.

This Panasonic Electric Bike wants to GO. It tries to pull off when you are stopped. Once you are going, you feel the smoothness of the integrated gears and silent motor start to take you away.

It is NOT one of those electric bikes where you pull the accelerator and you go like a motorbike. Not at all. You need to pedal, and once you are pedaling, your legs, the gears and the motor work together in perfect synchrony to move you, and move you FAST. But it is only a 250 W bike motor, so you will still be getting a lot of exercise, especially on the uphills. And of course if you want more exercise, all you have to do is turn the electric assistance level down to 1 or 0.

In terms of performance, I usually ride in the fastest 5% of cyclist commuters on my Panasonic Electric Bike. There ARE a few guys who pass me – couriers and super lean athletes on great road bikes. I am OK with that. I just want to get home in less than an hour and a half. On a regular bike, I usually just manage to keep up with the pack, because I have knee problems, and I am NOT super lean.

The other day I almost killed a guy – or I should rather say, he almost killed himself. He cut past me on a corner in that rude way that some (very rare) super fit cyclists do - just inches away from me, super fast and silent (not saying "On your left"), giving me a heck of a fright. Really rude. So I decided to just drop him on the next hill. Which I did, with a bit of effort and my Panasonic motor, leaving him in the dust. So he chased me down, and we got to a red light. I stopped, but this guy just zigzagged across four lanes of fast-moving traffic, scaring all the drivers and almost losing his life – just to prove he could drop me. Sad. Unfortunately, that kind of thing does happen occasionally when you ride a silent, high-performance electric bike. Usually, I let that kind of cyclist win, because I do not want to see them die.

Upgrades

I was not impressed by the quality or the size of the tires that came stock with the bike. But the wheel could accommodate a sturdier tire, so I upgraded from the stock Rubena 700 x 25 Syrinx tires to a set of Schwalbe Ultra Marathon Tires with Smart Guard (ordered online from Amazon!), which so far have lasted well and not had a single flat in a year of riding on urban streets. (Sometime in the future I will upgrade to better wheels, but right now, the stock wheels are working just fine.)

One advantage of upgrading to bigger tires is that it will take a bit of the shock out of the ride. This is a stiff bike, and so despite the carbon forks, I sometimes feel it in my wrists and elbows after a long ride. Bigger tires cushion the potholes on urban roads a bit.

I also upgraded the fender set, which originally was one tiny little decorative thing on the back wheel. For commuting, one needs good fenders that wrap right around the top of BOTH tires. The stock fender was more decorative than functional.

Also, note that unlike some other electric bikes, this one does not have integrated lights, so you will have to buy a set of lights (see my Average Joe Guide to Bike Lights).

I found the stock seat just fine. AND it looks good.

Durability of the Panasonic Electric Bike

I have been riding this bike hard for more than a year on tough roads. I have to admit that it is so slim and light that at first I was worried about whether it would hold up to my weight and speed. However, so far so good!

Bottom line on the Panasonic mid-drive bike motor on the Emotion BH E9502 Race Bike

I highly recommend this Panasonic electric bike, as well as this Panasonic bike motor on any decent bike. This is not a cheap option, but it's also not massively expensive. They go for around $3,000, and I managed to get mine on a sale for $2,000 from Evolution Bikes in North Vancouver.

Whether you pay $2,000 or $3,000, it is going to be excellent value for money.

Get this bike if you do long commutes and can't afford to spend three hours a day on a bike; or if your commute includes many long, grueling hills and you don't want to blow out your knees. Also if you just want to look like a super athlete on a handsome bike.

Technical Specs of the Emotion BH E9502 Race Bike

- Up to 62 miles of assisted cycling power per charge (not in my experience – the range is good, but not that good. Maybe at level 1 with the wind at your back, on flat ground ...)
- Smooth shifting Shimano 105 10 speed gear system (yes, awesome)
- Aluminum hydro-formed 28" Sport frameset (it hasn't broken yet, and I am heavy and ride it hard)
- Rubena 700 x 25 Syrinx tires (inferior tires for a bike this awesome – upgrade to something better before you even leave the shop)
- Removable battery pack with carrying handle (very handy and light)
- Perfect for racing or high performance sport riding (perfect for high performance sport riding, but you would obviously be disqualified if you tried to race with this kind of advantage!)
- 2 year warranty, extendable to 4 years (when I bought my bike you had to apply to the manufacturer for this rather than do it direct with the dealer, so I did not do it)

Guide to Bike Sizes

Bikes have sizes that are based on the height of the bicycle, measuring the length of the seat post tube. Some electric bikes, such as the Urbana (which has a BionX system) have geometry that is designed to fit all sizes.

However, most often you will need to know your bike size. You can figure out your bike size with the tables below. Of the two lengths (height and inseam), inseam is the most important.

Note: to make it a bit more complicated, there are different bike sizing systems. There's one system for road bikes, and then a different one that is used for mountain bikes and hybrid bikes. So first decide what kind of bike you want, then figure out your size, and you will be good to go!

Personally I have made the mistake of buying a bike that is too big, just because the price was right and I loved the bike. Big mistake! I could never get completely comfortable on the bike, and eventually I had to sell it. I hate to admit that I actually made this mistake twice! (I'm just a sucker for a pretty bike.) It's an expensive, time-wasting mistake, so don't do like I did, do like I say!

Start by knowing your bike size, and then double-check:

- Can you comfortably stand over the crossbar, without hurting any part of your body?
- Will you be able to stop safely, or will you have to fall gracelessly sideways until your feet make contact with the earth?

If the bike hurts you when you are standing over it, or is too big to stop safely, you will not have fun with the bike. Conversely, if the bike is too small, your knees and back will probably start to hurt, and you won't be able to deploy your body power efficiently (plus you will look funny!).

Adult Bike Sizes

Adult Hybrid and Mountain Bike Sizes

Your Height	Inseam Length	Bike Frame Size
4'11" to 5'3"	25" to 27"	13" to 15"
5'3" to 5'7"	27" to 29"	15" to 17"
5'7" to 5'11"	29" to 31"	17" to 19"
5'11" to 6'2"	31" to 33"	19" to 21"
6'2" to 6'4"	33" to 35"	21" to 23"
6'4" and up	35"	23"

Adult Road Bike Sizes

Your Height	Inseam Length	Bike Frame Size
4'10" to 5'1"	25.5" to 27"	46 to 48 cm
5'0" to 5'3"	26.5" to 28"	48 to 50 cm
5'6" to 5'9"	29.5" to 31"	52 to 54 cm
5'8" to 5'11"	30.5" to 32"	56 to 58 cm
5'10" to 6'1"	31.5" to 33"	58 to 60 cm
6'0" to 6'3"	32.5" to 34"	60 to 62 cm
6'2" to 6'5"	34.5" to 36"	62 to 64 cm

Height and Inseam

The tables above show bike sizes based on height and inseam. Note that for adults, inseam is the most important measurement, because it determines your standover height.

For example, a bike might be advertised as having a standover height of 27 inches. If your inseam is 29 inches, this means that you could stand up with this bike under you, and the cross bar would not damage your most delicate bits. (Obviously this is less important with step through style bikes that do not have a cross bar.)

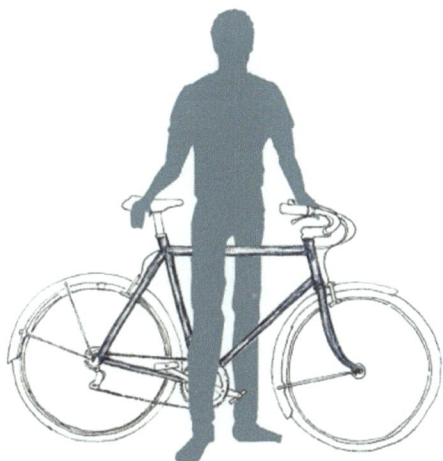

For road bikes you need to have about 1 to 3 inches of distance between the bar and your crotch; for mountain bikes you would be safer with a bit more (due to more bouncing and action on mountain trails).

Kid's Bike Sizes

Child's Age	Child's Height	Wheel Size
2 to 5	26" to 34"	12"
4 to 8	34" to 42"	16"
6 to 9	42" to 48"	18"
8 to 12	48" to 56"	20"
Youth	56" to 62"	24"

Guide to Bike Terminology

This list is intended for those fairly new to cycling, to help decipher terms that show up in adverts for bikes. Knowing the meaning of these terms will help you decide if you want to look at a particular bike. These terms apply to regular bikes as well as electric bikes.

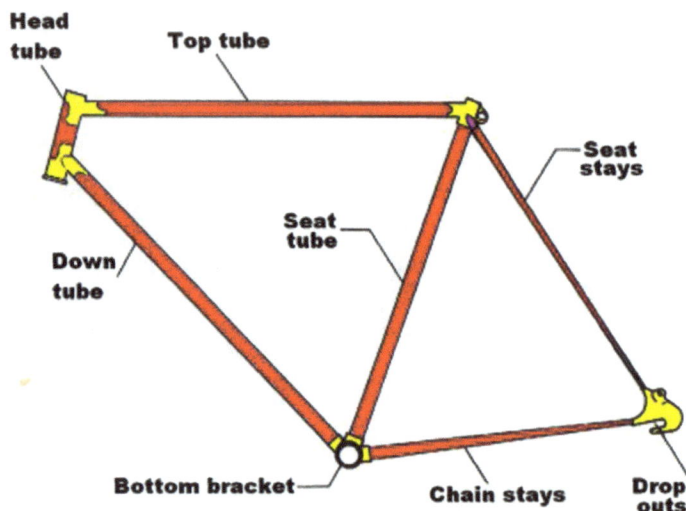

- **Aluminum bikes** – these have frames made of aluminum, which have become the default for most modern bikes. They tend to be lighter than steel bikes, and have fatter tubes.
- **ATBs** – all-terrain bikes – see Mountain bikes on p. 11.
- **BMX bikes** – bicycle motocross bikes, also called stunt bikes, used for tricks. Smaller bikes, with bare bones accessories, but often fitted with special equipment, such as pegs to stand on.
- **Bottom bracket** – the part to which the cranks attach.

- ☐ **Caliper brakes** – see **Rim brakes**, below.
- ☐ **Cantilever brakes** – see **Rim brakes**, below.
- ☐ **Carbon-fibre bikes** – these have frames made of carbon-fibre and are very light, but very expensive. They are not as strong as aluminum or steel. Some aluminum bikes do incorporate carbon parts. For example, carbon forks are fairly common on higher-end hybrids and road bikes, and are good at taking some of the edge off bumpy urban roads.
- ☐ **Components** – Refers to the pieces that are added to the frame to equip the bike, such as the gear system, brakes, shift levers, crank set and pedals, seatpost, handlebars and derailleurs. Better quality bikes have better quality components. An ad that says something like "top of the line components" indicates that the bike has better quality components. Of course, to be absolutely sure the seller is telling the truth you would have to research the components.
- ☐ **Cranks** – the part to which the pedals attach.
- ☐ **Chromoly** – Chrome Molybdenum Steel. A light, strong steel, often used to build fairly light, responsive, long-lasting frames. Sometimes called CRO MO.
- ☐ **Cruiser bikes or cruisers** – these usually

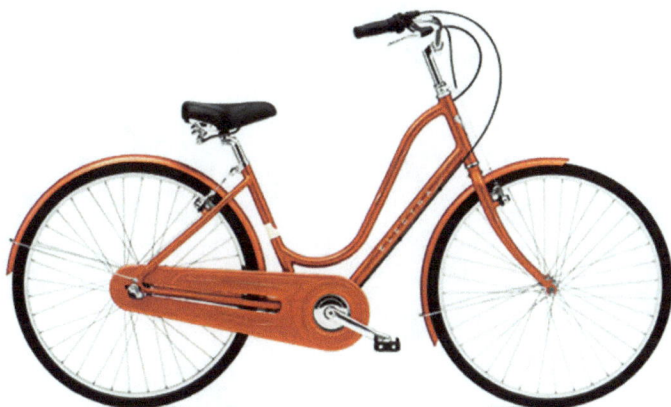

have balloon tires, upright seating posture, and single-speed drivetrains. They are pretty simple steel bikes, often incorporating quite stylish and fun designs. They are heavy but strong. They were very popular from the 1930s to the 1950s, and in recent times have become popular again. These are great bikes for riding in a leisurely way around a park, and they have many fans. In fact, if you live in a major city you might find a Cruiser Club you can join. However, personally I would not recommend them for commuting, touring or any kind of serious cycling.

☐ **Cyclocross bikes** – specialty bikes for cyclo-cross races. Much like road bikes, except the tires are fatter, and there are some other differences as well. If you don't know what they are, you probably don't need one (very few people do).

☐ **Derailleurs** – the name derailleurs comes from railway line derailleurs, because these are the things that move the chain from one chain ring onto the next. There are two of them, one at the front of the chain and one at the back. They are a high-maintenance part of the bike, needing frequent cleaning and oiling (like the chain). They are also very important to maintain – clean derailleurs will

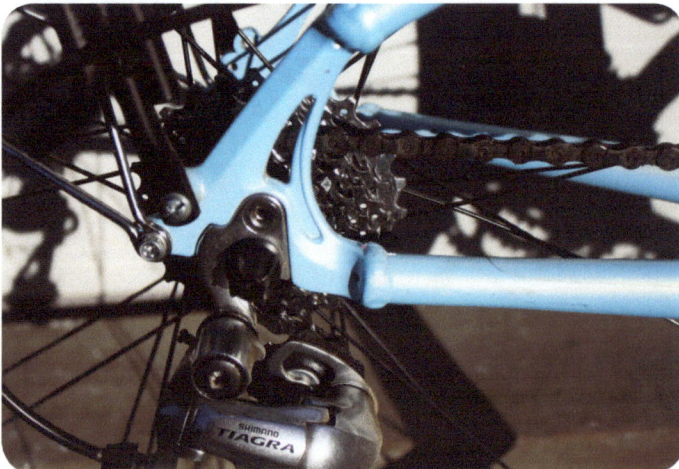

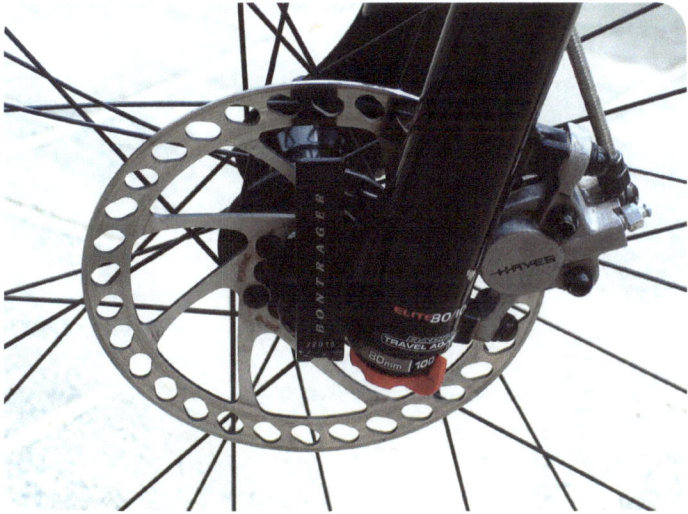

help keep your bike going well. I have a guide to a really easy way to keep your chain clean and lubed on my website at http://averagejoecyclist.com/how-to-keep-bike-chain-clean-lubed/

☐ **Disc brakes** – most commonly fitted to mountain bikes and electric bikes, disc brakes are heavier than other kinds of brakes. They work best with fat tires, and are almost never seen on road bikes. Basically they consist of a metal disc attached to the wheel hub. When the cyclist pulls on the brakes, pads squeeze the disc, slowing the wheel as kinetic (motion) energy is converted into thermal (heat) energy. There are two kinds of disc brakes: **hydraulic disc brakes** and **mechanical disc brakes.** Hydraulic disc brakes are considered superior. Personally I love hydraulic disc brakes on my electric bikes, as you need the braking power, as electric bikes are usually heavy and fast. and are especially useful when commuting in very wet weather. An alternative to disc brakes are Paul Motolite brakes, which also have amazing stopping power, but are caliper brakes.

☐ **Electric bikes** – bikes with electric assists, which make it easier to cycle up hill, and to cycle in general. Most of these offer a combination of pedaling and electrical assist, with the assist powered by a rechargeable battery. These bikes are wonderful as they make cycling more accessible for people who are older or who have physical ailments, such as knee problems. They also make it feasible for physically able people to commute long distances without excessive exhaustion or sweat. In fact, research indicates that people who buy electric bikes get fitter than people who buy regular bikes – simply because if you have an electric bike, you are more likely to use it for daily commuting.

☐ **Fixed gear bikes, also know as Fixies** – bikes that use a rear drive system, do not have a freewheel, and cannot coast. The pedals attach directly to the rear hub. Essentially you have to keep pedaling all the time, as these bikes usually have only a front brake, and sometimes have no brakes at all. When they have no brakes, you stop the bike by pedaling backwards. They usually only have one gear, as well. Why anyone would want one is beyond me, but if you do, please try before you buy, because they require a very different riding style. I remember I had one of these once, when I was a very little boy, and I recall having to brake by stamping down hard on the pedals. I was very happy to graduate to a real bike … However, these bikes are now considered to be very cool, so you can expect to pay more for them, even though they have less features.

☐ **Fork** – this is the part that houses the front wheel. It is attached to the main bike frame, and consists of two blades (most round, some flat) that travel downward to hold the front axle, thus allowing the cyclist to steer. Some have suspension built into them, others do not.

☐ **Frame prices** – the hierarchy of frame prices usually goes like this: low-end steel, low-end aluminum, low-end carbon, high-end aluminum, high-end steel and high-end carbon.

☐ **Full suspension bikes** – bikes with front and rear suspension. Many electric bikes now have full suspension (see also **Suspension**).

☐ **Hardtail** – a bike that has front suspension but does not have rear suspension.

☐ **Head tube** – the tube that contains the headset (steering bearings). The top and down tubes attach to this tube (see illustration on p. 4).

☐ **Hybrid bikes** – a cross between road bikes and mountain bikes, and a good choice for commuting in the urban jungle (see picture below). Not-so-young people sometimes find hybrids are easier on their backs. The tires are thinner than mountain bikes, but thicker than road bikes. (Tires can be changed, but only as much as the rims permit – for example, it is impossible to put a fat mountain bike tire on a thin road bike rim.) Hybrids have straight handlebars, and usually have a fairly upright riding position. Upright is good for riding in traffic, as you can see better. Bear in mind that riding position can be adjusted quite cheaply, by changing the handlebars or the riser (the part that attaches the handlebars to the frame.

☐ **Hydraulic disk brakes** – see **Disc brakes**.

☐ **Lug or Lugged (frame)** – some ads will proudly refer to a lugged frame. This refers to short angled tubes that are used to join and reinforce two or more tubes on a bicycle frame. They tend to make the bike frame stronger, and can look pretty good too. The vintage Bianchi frame above has lugs that are chromed, making them easier to see.

☐ **Mechanical disk brakes** – see **Disc brakes**.

☐ **Mixte/Step-through** – these bikes do not have a cross bar, making it easy to step on or off. They are sometimes called "lady's bikes," but in fact they are popular with all gender persuasions. They are especially useful if you have limited mobility, or are nervous because you haven't been on a bike for three or four decades. They are also great if you want to bike in a skirt.

☐ **Mountain bikes** – (also called all-terrain bikes or ATBs) bikes designed primarily for off road use, with straight handlebars, a strong (but heavier) frame, and fat (but again heavier) tires. Many have suspension shocks on the front, which add comfort (at the expense of weight). A feature I really like is suspension shocks with a lockout – this means you can turn off the shocks when you don't want or need them. Although these bikes are called mountain bikes, many never go off road, as they are also suitable for rough urban commuting. Bear in mind that their weight means you have to pedal harder for the same speed you could more easily achieve on a hybrid or a road bike. That's why, if you take a look at the flocks of urban cycle-commuters that are becoming increasingly common in modern cities, you will see far more road bikes than mountain bikes. The photo above shows what you could do with a mountain bike, but if you're not quite this athletic, don't worry – research shows that 95% of people who own mountain bikes **never** ride them on mountains, or even take them off road.

☐ **Pedelec** – a bike that also has an electric motor, which helps cyclists to pedal but does not replace pedaling.

☐ **Recumbent bikes (recumbents)** – bikes on which the seat is tilted back and low to the ground, usually with the pedals on top of the front wheel. Although it looks as if the rider is lying down, recumbent bikes are in fact said to be the fastest type of bike because they are so aerodynamic. Helpful for people with bad backs, too.

☐ **Rigid bike** – a bike with no suspension. Note this is not a bad thing – many of my favorite bikes are rigid! Suspension adds comfort, but it also adds weight, thereby decreasing cycling efficiency. It's also just another set of parts that can go wrong, and therefore just another set of parts that could be faulty on a used bike.

☐ **Rim brakes** – as the cyclist applies the brakes, friction pads apply braking force to the rims of the wheels, slowing the bike down. Rim brakes are cheap and easy to maintain, but are not great in wet weather (especially on steel rims). On the plus side, you can upgrade these kinds of brakes simply by buying better quality **brake pads**, which do not cost a lot of money. (Even if you buy a brand new bike, this is an area where manufacturers often save money by using low-quality pads, so even with a new bike you might want to upgrade the pads.) There are various kinds of rim brakes, including V-brakes, caliper brakes and cantilever brakes. **Caliper brakes** (below left) are self-contained, and are attached to the bike's frame with a single bolt. The arms reach downward and therefore need to be long enough to get around the tire. **Cantilever brakes** (below right) attach to the side of the frame or fork, requiring special brazed-on fittings on the frame. The brake consists of two separate arms, each of which is individually attached to the frame or fork. V-brakes developed from cantilever brakes, and are considered the most cost-efficient way to achieve powerful and

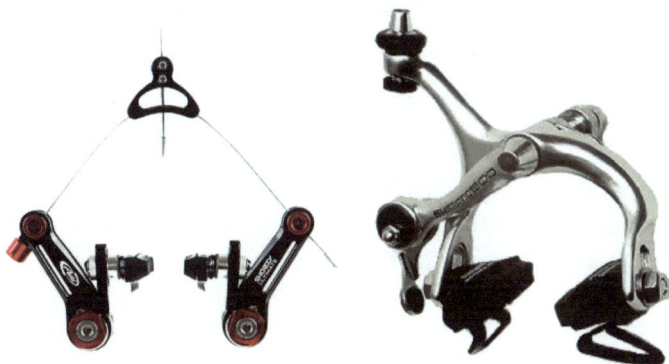

reliable braking. However, the older style cantilever brakes are well suited to the design of road bikes.

☐ **Road bikes (also called racing bikes)** – a lightweight bike with thin tires and (usually) drop handlebars, built for speed and a more aggressive style of cycling (your back is close to parallel to the road when your hands are in the drops). Although primarily built for racing, many people do use them for commuting. They are certainly the most efficient and fastest bikes.

☐ **Shimano** – countless ads will mention that the bike has "Shimano components" or "Shimano gears." This means that the bike's components or gears were made by a Japanese manufacturing company called Shimano. For your purposes, this means close to nothing at all.

Kinds of Shimano Components,
from highest to lowest quality

Mountain Bikes	Road, Hybrid, & Touring Bikes
XTR	Dura Ace Electronic
XT	Dura Ace
Deore LX	Ultegra
SLX (starting in 2009)	LX (starting in 2009)
Deore	105
Alivio	Alfine
Acera	Tiagra
Altus	Nexus
	Sora

Shimano has 50% of the world market in bicycle components, which means that they supply a full range of products, from bottom of the range to top of the range. A Shimano product could be close to garbage, or close to heaven. To find out which, use the tables supplied below. Or you can just ignore the allusion to Shimano, and examine other aspects of the bike. You can take a little comfort from the thought that as Shimano manufactures components for some of the world's greatest bikes, there must be some kind of positive trickle-down effect to the rest of its product line. (Shimano's primary competition are bicycle component manufacturers Campagnolo and SRAM).

The table will help you to figure out if a bike is a good buy, as it shows you the level of quality of various Shimano parts (top quality is at the top). The top levels are very expensive, and are mainly used on expensive race bikes; the average cyclist does not need the top levels. For example, Deore is good enough for the average cyclist's mountain bike – and Deore is only four levels from the bottom. In road bikes, the highest level I have ever owned is 105, and although I found those components awesome, I really did not need that level, as I am not even a casual racer. Tiagra and even Sora components are suitable for beginning and casual riders.

Bear in mind that if you have a very powerful engine on your bike, you will not use your gears much. I have spent a lot of time riding a 3-speed Pedal Easy bike, and the three gears were plenty, even with massive hills.

Note that there is one more level, right at the very bottom: Shimano parts with no model numbers or names; these are made for department store bikes, and are cheap and nasty. So just because the ad says "Shimano", this does not mean you are buying quality. Find out what kind of Shimano parts they are, and compare with the table to see where they fall.

- ☐ **Single speed** – these bikes only have one gear. They are popular at the moment, for reasons that escape me. My daughter wants one, which prompted me to ask her, "Why would you not take advantage of a century of advances in cycling technology?" To which her response was a withering look of pity, and a grunted "They're cool." I still think they're stupid, and they certainly make it hard to get up hills, or even to get the bike started. On the plus side, they're usually cheaper and lighter than geared bikes. And they don't have a geared derailleur system, so that is one less thing that can get dirty or broken – and one less thing that could be faulty on a used bike.

☐ **Steel bikes –** these have frames made of steel. Steel is a little heavier than some materials, but it is flexible and makes for a comfortable ride. Most older bikes are made of steel. There is nothing wrong with a steel bike – don't be taken in by the idea that you have to have an aluminum bike.

☐ **Suspension –** a system that suspends a cyclist so that the ride is not so bumpy. (See also **Hardtail** and **Full suspension bikes**, above.) Most common on mountain bikes, but also used on many hybrids. The suspension is most commonly built into the front fork, but may also be built into the rear of the bike, or the seat post or the hub. Mountain bikes with both front and rear suspension are becoming more common, and are referred to as full suspension bikes. Good ones are still very expensive. If you are buying a used full suspension bike, bear in mind that people who own these bikes often ride hard on rough terrain, or fearlessly hurtle down mountainsides, so the bike may have been soundly thrashed and possibly damaged. Check these even more carefully than regular bikes.

☐ **Touring bikes –** (also called Trekking bikes) bikes designed to handle the demands of cycle touring. Cycle touring by definition entails cycling long distances while carrying heavy loads, and touring bikes are adapted to facilitate this. For example, they may have a longer wheelbase, so that your heels do not bang into your saddle bags when pedaling (a very annoying thing). They are designed to be especially strong, and the frames have several mounting points so that multiple panniers and luggage holders can be carried. They are usually designed for comfort as well, given that bike tourists may spend many hours of the day in the saddle. Many cyclists are now using electric bikes for touring, for the obvious reason that they extend your range. Of course, you need a very good battery, because you don't want to be out of battery power with a heavy, loaded bike somewhere in the Alps!

☐ **Trailer bikes** – a bike that is trailed along by another bike in front. A tow bar hooks it to the bike that is pulling it. The trailer bike just has a back wheel, a seat, pedals and handlebars for the young rider to hold on to. These are designed for younger riders so that they can safely join their parents on rides. Of course it is much easier to tow someone with an electric bike, so an increasing number of parents are getting their children to school using electric bikes with trailers.

☐ **V-brakes** – these were developed by Shimano from cantilever brakes. V-brakes are a side-pull version of cantilever brakes and, like cantilever brakes, are mounted on the frame. V-brakes or disc brakes are best for mountain bikes. The photo of V-brakes is from the website http://sheldonbrown.com/home.html – a great resource for the cycling community, generously created by the late, great Sheldon Brown. Check it out if you want to learn much, much more about bikes.

If you find this guide useful, you might also like:

Average Joe Cyclist's Bike Buyers Guide

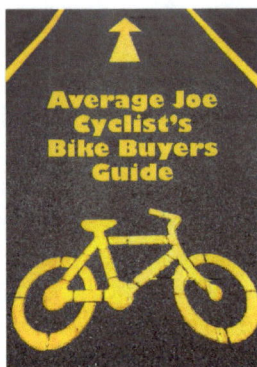

Extraordinary Recipes: How We Lost Weight by Eating Well

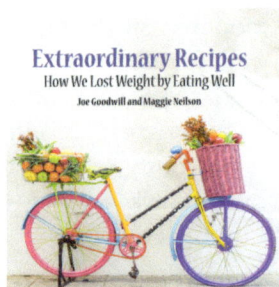

Average Joe Cyclist Blog

Tons of free information at http://averagejoecyclist.com/

Ride On!